A NIGHT IN JAIL

A Novella

By

H.A. Swan and K. Anderson

A story about drugs and mental illness, inspired by true events

ISBN: 978-0-692-96707-2

Book layout by www.ebooklaunch.com

Cover by Karen Phillips/PhillipsCovers.com

ACKNOWLEGEMENTS

I'd like to begin by thanking our family. To Glenda Anderson, our mother. Your expert critiques and endless belief helped and motivated me. No one can write a synopsis with dash and flair like my mom! To Robert D. Anderson, our father. Your generosity and encouraging words are deeply appreciated. To our sisters: Rachelle, for illustrating the big picture for me when I cannot see it; and Crystal, for being an enthusiastic reader.

To Christine and Jackie who advised me to write a book they would want to read, not a book they should read.

Fond appreciation to my writers' group: Jalé, Sandi, and Jennifer.

Big thanks to my friends, Jamie, Robin and Janet for reading and rooting me onward.

My Toastmasters Club: Your feedback affirmed the messages of this book and the writer/speaker who was telling them.

To Steve from Power Ten Web Design, for your prodigious skills, effort and ongoing good humor.

Thank you to the King County Department of Adult and Juvenile Delinquency Records Department for providing the mug shots which tell their own stunning story.

To Christopher J. Lynch, author of several entertaining books, your guidance through the self-publishing process made my life so much easier.

K. is grateful to Gary, Dr. James Tracy, and Priscilla, for their enduring friendships.

To my stepson, Connor: your astute observations and suggestions greatly improved the story. To my son, Nick, thank you for making me laugh.

And most of all, to Joe: the rock from which my flower grows. Yes, I'm lucky you love me!

DEDICATION

My brother lived the life of a homeless, mentally ill, repeatedly incarcerated drug addict and dealer - but he was not alone in his suffering. Our whole family agonized helplessly for many, many years. In order to shed a light on its tormenting issues, our parents and siblings gave their whole-hearted support in the telling of this story.

With our deepest gratitude, K and I dedicate this novella to our family.

H.A. Swan

"You can outdistance that which is running after you
but not what is running inside you."

-A Rwandan proverb

Police Department

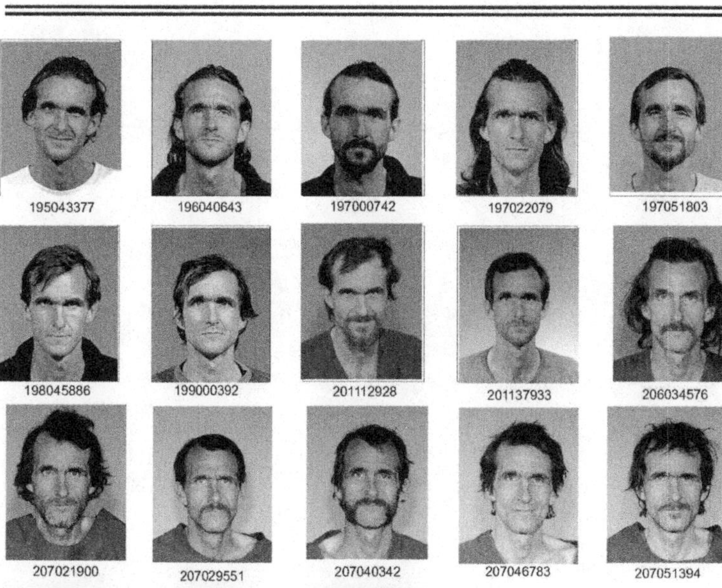

Seattle 1978

Saturday night

9:39 PM: The guard clamps his beefy-fisted grip around my arm, pulling me toward the cell. He's enjoying my humiliation way too much. He acts like he never got drunk or high when he was eighteen. Like I believe that for one second. I know he must have had fun once in his life. He should cut me some slack. Christ, my parents should cut me some slack.

I do not belong in there. This is ridiculous! Everyone I know is doing it! One day, marijuana is going to be legalized and this "punishment" will all be for nothing.

On the phone, my dad was pissed. He said his professional reputation was at stake because of my behavior. My mom blathered on and on about how disappointed she was in me. She was crying. I couldn't handle all their drama.

Reality Rush.

That's what I call it. When the car is thick with pot smoke, I'm on an amazing high, filling another bowl, laughing with my friends. But then a bright light — the flashlight from a police car — suddenly cuts through the hazy smoke and I gotta come down fast, straighten up and deal with reality.

Reality Rush Number Two: my parents refused to bail me out. My best friends' parents came to pick them up from the police station! But my parents said a night in jail will do me some good. Teach me some kind of bullshit lesson. The guards took away my clothes. I got fingerprinted, photographed, and put in a jumpsuit. They treated me like an ax murderer.

Two Reality Rushes in one night means a third one has to be coming, because Bad Things Come in Threes. What's next?

I dig my feet in as Officer Beef drags me closer to the cell door. Maybe if I go right to sleep I can prevent the other bad thing from happening. I just need to make it through until tomorrow morning. Tomorrow morning! God, it feels as far away as next year.

"What if my parents post bail right now? Can I get out early?"

"Nope. Yer paperwork ain't in so yew missed early release. Ya git out with ever' body else at 8:00 AM."

Jerk. I'll bet these dudes dip into our stash when they confiscate it.

9:43 PM: Officer Beef yanks me over the threshold. I am now in hell. Christ, it stinks like an outhouse in here. Maybe the toilet against the wall doesn't flush or something. Even though I'm stoned, it still hits me how this looks exactly like what you see on TV, except without any bars. Names, dates, and gang signs are written all over the concrete walls and steel beams. A huge window separates the jail cell from Beefy's station, so he can watch my every move. Other than the toilet, there's only one place to sit down. It's a steel bench. And someone's sleeping on it already.

I keep an eye on the clock hanging on the guard's wall. The hands tick extra slowly, like we're in a *Twilight Zone* episode. Each hand hoists a ball and chain that weighs me down and holds me back from being freed from this dungeon.

God, I can't breathe. Officer Beef doesn't seem to notice or care. I cover my nose and look at the guy on the bench again. Man, that is definitely where the piss smell is coming from. He is single-handedly humidifying the room with his stench. He's a homeless dude.

I plead with the officer, "Where am I supposed to sleep? There's only one bench?"

"Thassright." Beef tightens his grip, he won't let go.

Homeless has long, thin, scraggly hair that's balding on top; he looks like the butler in *The Rocky Horror Picture Show.* His knobby, skinny claws hold a flattened roll of toilet paper under his head. His fingers are long and, like his whole body, covered with a film of dirt. Maybe the police dredged him out of a sewer. He smells like puke too. I can't sleep unless I've showered because I can't stand my own B.O. I hold my sleeve over my nose like a gas mask.

Officer Beef punctuates my perp walk with an unnecessary shove. I trip and land on the concrete floor. Right on my knees. Shit. It hurts like hell, but I don't want to let him have another laugh at my expense.

"Come on, you didn't have to…"

"Keep smokin' pot and you'll ruin yer basketball skills. An' everythin' else."

What? I rub my knees and turn to look at his fleshy face from the cold floor.

"Yer team played against my son's team las' month." He motions to his own fat, clean-shaven cheek. "I remember yer sideburns and yer lay-ups."

My sideburns are the reason the coach won't advance me to the A-team. "My friends were doing it, not me. I don't smoke pot!"

"Sure ya don't." Beefy leaves, shaking his head.

"Officer, where are the blankets?"

Beefy slams the door shut with a CLANK!

Suddenly, Homeless leaps up from the bench. Oh shit! I scramble right back up to my feet! His hair sticks out. His eyes bulge at me. He shouts: "WHAT? OH MY GOD!"

9:47 PM: He's one of those bat-shit-crazy people you see outside all the time. His red, creased eyes grow even wider. Homeless grips his heart like I've scared him to death. He heaves, "Who are you?!"

"Dude, it's okay. Calm down."

"What do you want?"

"Nothing!"

"Bullshit! You — you — holy shit!" He looks lost.

"You're in jail. The guard woke you. You're in jail."

"You're fucking with me! You're messing with my head!"

"I told you it wasn't me! It was the guard!"

"Who are you? What's your name?"

"Danny."

"Fuck you 'it's Danny'!" His hands shake.

He steps toward me. I jerk back; I'm shaking too. I can't fight — I'm high! Where do I go? I spin around and bang on the guard's window.

Beef has his back to me. I scream, "Hey, Officer! He's crazy! Help!! Help me!! He's crazy!!"

Beef glances at me. Bored. Can't he see what's happening? Beef blinks. He bites a sandwich. He brushes the breadcrumbs and my pleas, like dandruff, off his shirt. He's not doing shit.

Oh, man. No. No way. I cannot be stuck in here all night long with this crazy person. I swallow. I turn back around to Homeless.

9:50 PM: He moves closer. Red face. Jugular veins. "You're following me, Danny."

"I'm not."

"All of you. For years! Now this? This is science fiction! How did you fuckers do it?" I back away from him, bumping against the glass wall.

I shudder to my core. I stare straight into his popping, bloodshot eyes. "Dude, I didn't do anything!"

"Are you real?" He comes closer.

No! I cross my arms over my face and cover my head. "Don't touch me!" He touches my forearm. I jerk away. "Back off, I mean it!!" Avoid a fight. Avoid a fight. That's what they say. I peek through my arms.

"Oh God." He steps back; his hand is over his mouth. "What…what are your parents' names?"

"Ted and Cara."

"Cara? Cara what? What's her maiden name?"

"Whittaker."

"Cara Whittaker. Cara Whittaker. Ted what?"

"What?"

"Your last name! What's your last name?"

"Oh. Oh. It's Johnson!"

"Danny Johnson? You expect me to believe that bullshit?"

"Look, I don't know who you think I am — or what you think I'm doing — but I am not following you!"

"Yeah? Prove it!" He blasts. "Prove it!!"

"Okay — okay! I'll prove it to you; I won't talk to you!" I edge to the corner. "I swear to God. I'm not following you! I don't know who you are. And I don't care, man. I'm telling you — I don't care!" I slide down to the floor and make myself as small as possible. I hold my hands up. "See? I'm really sorry I woke you. You can go back to sleep, okay?"

"You think I'm stupid?! I'm not sleeping in front of you! Who knows what crazy shit you'll do to me!" Jesus. That's exactly what I'm thinking about him.

He points his leathery claw at me. "Stay there. I command you to stay in that corner. So I can watch you."

9:59 PM: In junior high, I read a book which said I should make a list of my life goals to stay on track. So I did it. It may sound corny, but ever since that day I've carried that list with me everywhere I go. It's soft and faded and almost falling apart because it's gone through the laundry so many times. It says:

1. Become a lawyer
2. Get married
3. Become a great skier

Instinctively, I touch my hip, feeling for my list. Of course, my list isn't on me; it's in the front pocket of my jeans. I checked it in with the rest of my clothes when they issued me this jumpsuit.

Homeless snatches up the toilet roll that unraveled all over the floor. As he paws it back up with his yellow fingernails, he paces the small space like a caged, rabid animal. He mumbles, "Ted Johnson…Cara Whittaker Johnson."

He stares at me. His weathered and lined face sags over his global Adam's apple. His whiskers spring out of the dirt yard around his mouth like dead weeds. He repeats the names over and over.

Those are not my parents' names. And my name isn't Danny. I pulled them all out of my ass. I won't tell him one damn thing. Maybe he could come find me after he gets out and burn down our house or my dad's new apartment. I'd never hear the end of it. But then it would be my parents' own damn fault for making me stay here.

Will Crazy kill me? Will he gouge my eyes out with his knobby fingers? Kick me to death? Strangle me with his ropy hair? I wedge myself into my corner as far as I can possibly go. I pull my jumpsuit away from my chest so he can't see my pounding heartbeats. I size him up: he's as tall as me. His wrists are skinny and look like they've been shrunk wrapped in brown paper. I could snap his arms in half if he comes at me.

He confronts me. The veins pulse out of his neck. "What do you want from me?"

"Actually — I — I do want something from you. Just one thing."

"What?! What is it?!"

"I want to ignore you, okay? That's the truth! One hundred percent! And I'm really good at ignoring people. I do it to my parents all the time!"

He's stunned. It looks like I clonked him in the forehead with my frisbee. Then, with sudden bursts, he laughs. "Ha! Ha, ha, ha!" He totters back a step and beams at me, "Good one!"

He thinks this is funny? I'm having a fucking heart attack. I try to catch my breath. Christ, at least I found a way to keep him from killing me.

10:01 PM: He sits on the bench. He eyes me over his long nose hairs that jut out like whiskers. He inspects me the way my mom does when she thinks I might be high. "On a sacred oath, you really don't know who I am?"

"No! I don't!" I put up my hand. "And I don't want to know!"

"Ha, ha!" His stupid grin gives me an unwelcome peek at his swollen gums. They're red and black and losing their grip on his five remaining teeth. Yeah, it's exactly like what you see at the dentist where they try to scare you into flossing. He cackles, "You're funny! Ahhh…I needed a laugh. Besides, you and your parents have twelve letters in your first names when you combine them. Twelve is a biblical number. Twelve disciples, twelve tribes. So that's a good sign. Name is Captain."

Ugh. No — No, no, no, no. No introductions. I wish he'd let me pretend to sleep so I don't have to talk to him. But no, he keeps gumming, "I didn't mean to scare you. It's just you — this — this is so — I've never imagined they would go this far! But here we are — in jail. This is my eighteenth time here."

My jaw drops.

He laughs, "Ha! Ha! Your face! Don't be frightened, Grasshopper! I'm not violent. Just drugs. Today, I got arrested because I didn't pay attention to the signs. If I get busted one more time, it's three strikes and I'm out. I'll be sent to prison. Not just jail. Prison. Fucking no way. That would be part of their grand ploy to put me away for good so they can watch me more closely. They'd love that. More free entertainment for them at my expense. But it is serious shit. If I go to prison, I'll get parole and then I'll get tested for drugs on a regular basis. I can't survive the streets without alcohol or drugs. Eventually, I'll test positive. Then I'll be back in prison in a cycle that will never end. I can't go to prison, Danny. Jail is easy. Jail is just juvenile boot camp."

"It is?"

"Yes! So cool the fuck down! All that yelling and screaming at the guard and banging on the window is going to make it worse for you. The guard's just doing his time like you and me. If you need anything you're supposed to send a *kite*."

"What? A what?"

"You write down what you want on a piece of paper and send it. A kite."

Captain lumbers over to a holder on the wall where there's some paper and pencils. He points out a slot which is right next to it. "You put it in here. They'll pick it up when they fucking feel like it. Could be hours from now. But they don't like it when you summon them like they're your servants."

"I just wanted to..."

"Think about how hard it would be to work here!" He waves at the walls. "This place is drab. It's sad. Know what? The exact same guy did my intake like four or five times in a row. Down here? Where there's no windows? Danny, the brightest thing he had to look at all day long was our jumpsuits. But when they get a job as a jailer, they stick with it. Stay trapped underground with inmates for twenty years, waiting it out to get their benefits and retirement. All so the public can stay at home and watch TV. So think about that before you write your kite."

"Uh, okay." I don't want to encourage him. But I'm curious. "Why do they call it a kite?"

"They could call it a piece of shit. Who knows? The process is the punishment. You're used to getting immediate answers, but in jail, you won't get a yes or no. You could be in this cold cell with a bunch of other people and you're not comfortable and you have to wait and not hit anybody. Locked in a room with ten other guys who think the world owes them something. Like I said, I'm a nice guy, Danny, anybody else comes in here, you don't want to come at them with your sense of humor because — *BAM!*" He punches his fist in his palm. I jump. "You're going to get hit. And if we got trouble, the guards won't rush in. Coming in contact with the homeless is the worst part of their job because we're not checked for scabies or lice and, just like everybody else, the guards don't want to bring anything home. No credit cards accepted, especially if you're here for twenty-four hours. We could be stuck in here with standing room only. Just standing and breathing with ten other angry dudes. It's a big deal here to get a bed roll and a bench. God help anybody that uses the toilet. Plus, if you complain about something the guards could decide to keep you here longer. To punish you for as long as they want! Look, kid, with the guards, all you want to do is to earn *Happy Time.*

That's when you're getting movement and they're facilitating it. But you can't be complaining at them and pounding on the windows."

Holy shit.

10:06 PM: I need a toke…right now. I can't take this guy while I'm high. But no way will I be able to handle all his insanity when I sober up. In a jail cell that smells like a bus station urinal. Plus, I'll have to deal with how bad this is. I'm eighteen and this is going on my record. Sure as hell hope this doesn't mess up my chances to go to law school or pass the bar.

Another corny truth about me: I didn't know I would have to go to college before I went to law school. I was totally amped to go and get my law degree right after high school graduation. But then my parents informed me it doesn't work like that. It's funny to think about now but, a couple years ago, I was really disappointed.

Hopefully my parents will inform me that a night in jail won't hurt my future; that it doesn't work like that. That my arrest will appear as innocently as a few parking tickets. Just handle the paperwork, move on, and no one in college or law school needs to know. But I can't think too far ahead. I have to focus on getting Happy Time.

I notice Captain's not saying anything. I look up. He's blinking and smiling at me, like I'm a kitten or something. "Funny we were talking about kites, because you're high as a kite, aren't you?" He sings, "*Rrrr-ocket Man!*"

"I'm not. I'm cold. I need a blanket."

"Good! Don't incriminate yourself! But yeah, yeah, yeah you're high. I mean, who the hell do you think you're talking to, anyway, Danny Johnson? Haven't you heard you shouldn't bullshit a bullshitter? After all my years in jail, rehab, AA, NA, and working the streets, I can tell a crackhead to a speedhead, a junkie to an acidhead, or a drunk to a stoner. And you, Danny, are stoned."

"Look, I'm not..."

"Danny, I get it. Getting high is a sacrament to a higher power. I know! It's a very intense way of capturing everything God has to offer. When I'm on the street, I'm sure I'm ready for whatever He brings my way. A car might drive up next to me and invite me inside. They could whisk me off to a new life with a home and a wife and kids. But for me to be ready for a miracle of that magnitude, I need my crack. So I'm totally with ya on getting high. But the problem is you are so stoned right now you don't realize what the holy fuck is going on in here. With me. And you." Captain leans toward me, fuming in my face. He hisses, "You have no idea. Do you?"

Something twinges on the back of my neck. Like the furry and tiny scratches of a baby rodent. Is this dungeon infested? Flecking the back of my hair, I don't find anything. I scan the cell for any kind of creature or bug. Nothing.

Pulling back from Captain, I hold my breath and pinch my lips together tight. I mutter, "I don't know what you're talking about."

"I mean in all the seventeen other times I've been hauled into this jail, I have never been in a cell with just one other person." He points his nose to the clock in the guard's room. "See the time?"

10:10 PM: I move away from Captain. Suck in some clean air and look at the clock. "It's ten after ten?"

"Exactly! It's 10:10! How do you think you and me just happened to wind up in here together? All by ourselves? Just you and me. At 10:10?" He tilts his head and whispers: "You are dumber than you look if you think this is just a coincidence."

10:11 PM: "There is no way we're the only two people under arrest in Seattle, Washington tonight. They probably put a whole van full of guys in the library or somewhere else."

"I've never been in jail so..."

"You ever notice that every time you see an ad for a watch, the hands are at 10:10?"

"Uh, no I didn't."

"'Friends, Romans, countrymen, lend me your ears!' 'Friends': one syllable. 'Romans': two. 'Countrymen': three. 'Lend me your ears': fourth in the list! And four syllables! These are practical implications with numbers. Judas was the thirteenth disciple. There are buildings made without the thirteenth floor! 10:10 is a time that advertisers consistently pay for! It is real! Real! Any triple digit number is biblical, Danny. Don't forget that. A triple-digit number means you should beware. And 10:10 means you should pay attention. Numerology gives you the ability to crack the code that will get you everything you want. Put you at the right place at the right time. Change your existence entirely. Every number has significance. Even if there's a number that's insignificant, that fact by itself, gives significance to that number."

It's ridiculous he pays so much attention to numbers. And the ones on the clock! What's all this crap prove? Even a broken clock is right two times a day. Must have been all the drugs.

"So?"

He points his finger to the ceiling. "That's a sign! Like I already told you, I ignored a sign — a very important sign — and I got arrested. You understand? The numbers are telling you to pay attention, Danny. Are you paying attention to them? I'm in jail tonight because I ignored the warning the numbers were giving me this morning — I really blew it!"

I mouth, "Ah".

"It started out as a normal day. Nothing out of the ordinary except it was sunny. Rare. A sunny day in Seattle. I was at my regular spot where I've always dealt drugs. My perch on The Ave. You been to the U District?"

That's a busy area by the University of Washington where I'm starting school next month. Maybe he'll tell me something useful about scoring pot there so I'll pay attention. I say, "Once or twice."

"Are you going to college?"

I lie, "I'm going to Wazzu." That's what we call Washington State University, a school in Pullman. I said that because it's several hours away and I don't want him looking for me in the U District. I off-handedly ask, "So what's happening on The Ave?"

Captain takes a pencil out of the holder on the wall. He taps it on his palm like a cigarette on its pack. "The Ave is two blocks in the University District. It's got all kinds of shops, restaurants, espresso houses, bars, and bookstores. Those blocks are hopping, not just with college kids like you, but with the miserable people of society who are just trying to figure out how they will survive the day. People are off their hinges. Mentally-ill people who talk to themselves, the guys on Social Security who live in boarding houses and have nowhere to go, the homeless teens scraping by, the do-gooders going into one of several churches, and the dealers. It's the dealers, like me, who own The Ave."

Captain lifts one eyebrow at me, letting me know how cool his job is. I side nod my head, as though I agree with him. I say, "Yeah?"

He puts the pencil behind his ear and continues, "So this morning, a fat guy was eyeballing me, all freaked out, not carrying any shopping bags, or eating, or anything. I could tell he wasn't a cop because he looked like a potato in his shirt sleeves. Dopey. Undercover cops try to look sharp, act sharp. He was so skittish, the second time he walked past my perch, he tripped. He might as well have had a flashing sign over his combed-over head announcing he was looking to buy something. Whatever substance he wanted, I was the right guy to sell it to him. See, he already passed up some other dealers a few doors down. They were clustered together, loud and laughing in their flashy clothes. He was right to steer clear of them. They probably would've laughed at him and they would've definitely stolen his money. I'm a lone guy, much older than anyone else, so I'm a lot less threatening to someone unfamiliar with this business. I asked him what he was looking for. He pushed up his horn-rimmed glasses and shifted in his feet, trying to act cool, which this dweeb will never be."

"What did he want?"

"Forty bucks worth of pot." Captain puts his foot on the toilet seat, rests an elbow on his knee. "I had a guy at a coffee shop down the street with a backpack full of weed. Earlier, when I first got on the block, I checked out the situation: who was selling, who had what for how much; who was offering me a good deal. I knew who had good stuff and who didn't. Sage, the dealer with the backpack, said he'd sell me eighth of an ounce for thirty bucks. So I tell my new customer to give me forty, plus another ten when I have it done. That way, I have ten for crack and ten for a burger and chocolate shake. I told my new client to give me his cash and I'd bring him back his drugs. This made him suspicious, but I was used to that and didn't take it personally. I was about to walk off with his money and possibly never return. In the past, I've had to leave my Washington State ID with some customers who were afraid to trust me. Talk about ridiculous! I could've lost my ID so they wouldn't lose forty bucks or whatever. Anyway, it wound up I did get my ID back. So, I had to give this potato my regular pitch."

"Did you get him his pot?"

"I'm getting to that." Captain leans against the wall and holds the pencil like a lit cigarette. "My pitch goes like this,

'Look, I'm here because no one is looking for me…' Then, all of a sudden, Sylvia, a street drunk, stumbles up to us and yells, 'DON'T TRUST HIM! He's the craziest fucker out there!' Now, let me tell you, Danny, this was ironic because she's the crazy one. Every day, she's got eyeliner smeared across half her face with lopsided bed head. So she snuggles up next to me, waving her cigarette, and goes, 'You don't want to deal with his crazy ass!' She laughed so hard she was hacking her morning-Menthol-beer-breath in our faces. The next thing I knew, my new client was looking around to see if he had any better choices. Which, like I told you already, he did not. I finally got her to take her coughing fur balls somewhere else but not before she elbowed me in the ribs. Funny for her, but she didn't need to make my life any harder. I told her I wouldn't ever buy her a beer again."

"So then you went to find Sage?"

Captain sits on the edge of the toilet seat and points his pencil at me. "Yes. But I'm telling you all this so you'll understand why I made the decision I did later on. Getting my new client to trust me was hard enough, like I explained. But Sylvia made it that much harder for me. So I looked my potential new client square in the eyes, right through his dandruff-flecked glasses. I'm always nice, but I had to go the extra mile here to be sure I showed how much I cared about good customer service. So I had to really sell myself and I said, 'Sylvia's just messin' around. You can tell, right? I mean, look. I can sit here in broad daylight because I don't have to hide from any pissed-off dealers or unhappy customers. That's because I always do a fair deal and everyone can trust me. I can get you what you want.' I treated every customer like he was going to be a return customer. And I loved it when I saw a familiar face, because then I knew I didn't have to go through all that again. My sales pitch seemed to make sense to him and he gave me his money. I told him I'd be out of sight with his cash, but I'd be back in a few minutes. I hopped off my perch. And that's when I saw it."

Agitated, Captains stands up.

"What?"

"A lottery ticket." He writes the numbers 999 on the wall. "The numbers 999! The ticket was practically waving at me from inside the garbage can!" Captain impels the pencil back in its wall holder, angry. He sees I don't get the 999 thing and sighs. "Danny, if you flip them upside down it's a sign of The Beast. 666!"

"Oh."

"The Beast?! How can you not care about 666? That's biblical! Lucifer!? That was my warning I should be careful." He stomps his foot. "Danny, if you were given a severe warning that something bad was going to happen, what would you have done?"

"I dunno…"

"What I should have done was return the money to my new client and go hide out somewhere for the rest of the day. But no. What I did was, I pulled my hood tighter around my face and quickly, yet very cautiously, continued on my way to Sage. I knew I had to make my new customer happy or I would never see him again. And I hadn't had my crack yet so I had to feed my craving. So, then, Jedda Jay, a dealer I work with, stopped me. His pals were dancing and working out a routine together because they think they'll graduate from The Ave to become musical sensations. I spot checked all corners to see if anyone was watching us. Nobody. Jedda slipped me a baggie with a little piece of crack in it. It was a gift from him to get me started for the day. I really appreciated it. I needed it! I really fucking needed it! He knew I was the only middleman on The Ave who was a crack addict. His good business acumen made me want to bring him a lot of customers. But at the same time, this confused me. I was warned by the three numbers — but

Jedda Jay's gift made me think it could be a good day. I don't like contradictory messages. It's confusing. Anyway, I went behind a dumpster and got high really fast."

Captain stretches like an actor arising from bed in a mattress commercial. His face alights with glory. "Danny, to come out from behind the dumpster and see The Ave...People bustling! The traffic! Sounds! It's just magical! To be a part of the city is magic!" He cherishes the sensory experience. "Feeling that good, I went on my way to get the pot from Sage."

Sage. I sit up. Time to pay attention. I ask, "Which coffee shop?"

"I'll tell you later, Rocket Man. Suddenly, this guy in an expensive tan leather jacket bee-lined to me. Under his breath, he said, 'What are you selling?' Now, my customer was waiting for his weed. But I didn't want to pass up a chance to have a new client with a lot of money. But something about this guy felt wrong. He was too direct, too slick. Maybe undercover. But his shined shoes matched his buttery jacket. And he wasn't giving me any bullshit about how to do the transaction like Mr. Potato Head. Jedda's gift showed me the day was going to be a lucky day, so I asked the guy what he wanted. He said he wanted crack. But his thumb didn't have a callous from holding a lighter open. I knew it was iffy. Then he pulled out $200. Not only would I have had enough money to go back to my camp and light candles and play cards the rest of the day, but I would've had enough to start the next day with a hit of crack. What would you have done, Danny?"

"Gone to Sage."

He shrugs, "Well, you're a pot head." I fake smile. He continues, "But I took his money and told him to stay right there. I ran back to Jedda, bought the crack, stashed half of it in my own pocket, and returned to Buttery Leather Jacket who was waiting patiently, smoking a cigarette. I made professional eye contact, gave him my engaging smile and I told him I hoped to see him again. He held out his hand to take the baggie. But I always did a controlled buy: it went on the railing. I turned and left. Now, I had to get my other deal done really, really quickly. As I hustled to the coffee shop, I was thinking about what a great day it had turned out to be when — BAM!"

Captain smacks his hands in front of my face. I flinch and say, "Hey!"

"That's how shocked I was too! I got tackled to the ground — face first! I was under arrest. Leather Jacket was an undercover cop. See, Danny? If I had heeded the warning, I would not be here tonight." He pauses. "Now, do you see my point? The time of 10:10 was telling you, Danny, that you need to pay attention."

"Oh..."

"So, are you paying attention?" He folds his arms and leans against the wall. "Because they are listening to us right now."

"To us? Who?"

"You've heard of where a guy gets convicted because he squawks to his cellmate?"

"Yeah."

"So, for a newbie, you're doing a good job of keeping your trap shut. Keep it that way, so whatever you say isn't used against you. Me? I've been in jail so many times, everything about me is public knowledge so who gives a shit. But right now, tonight, they are listening to me because they want to hear what I have to say to you." He goes to the guard's window. "And they're watching us."

I roll my eyes. "Isn't that what the window is for?"

"Of course the guard's watching us, you teenage asshole. I mean *The Others*. The Others you obviously don't have any clue about. They're watching us through hidden cameras." His eyes dart around the room. Still at the guard's window, he pads his fingertips along the outer part of its frame like he's reading Braille.

Beefy doesn't look up from his monitors. He must know Captain, or be used to people acting like freaks. I sigh, "Hidden cameras?"

"They're spying on me for their personal enjoyment because I'm Chosen. Now, it would appear, so are you."

10:41 PM: Chosen for what? And am I supposed to act like I care? Over the last few minutes he's walked over all the walls and floor with his fingers, and has kept babbling on and on and on about who-the-fuck knows what. I have no clue if he's found anything, but I'm losing my patience for his constant walking and talking in circles.

In that whole stupid story about getting arrested, he didn't tell me where to find the guy who has the backpack full of pot. Captain has taught me one important thing: he has absolutely nothing of value to say. So I've completely stopped listening to him.

Was he a ranting lunatic and then he became homeless, or did he lose his mind because he was homeless? How did he become homeless in the first place? He's obviously not dumb. He must've done a shitload of bad things to wind up like this. I see homeless people all the time and it seems like they've always been on the street. It's like they're a different human species, like Neanderthals or something. Not quite like the rest of us.

This guy must not have parents or family that give a flying fuck about him because if he did, there's no way they'd let him live outside. I've slept outside plenty of times. But we were camping. It was supposed to be for fun. Did he even have a mother and father? Was he ever taken to Boy Scouts or taught how to ski? Maybe his mom didn't fix him homemade whole wheat cinnamon rolls for breakfast or make him eat vegetables every day like mine did. Maybe he didn't go to a good school or was taken to church four times a week. Maybe he didn't get good grades or rock at speech and debate the way I do. He must have been neglected as a child. Maybe if he had a decent upbringing like me, he could have turned out better.

He probably didn't have a goal to be anything other than a druggie. I wonder if sleeping in jail is a step up for him. At least he has a roof over his head and a roll of toilet paper underneath it.

Captain's on his knees feeling along the bottom of the bench. He drones on, "If you had a radio and a TV, you'd tune them so they would be in sync. It's the same with life: you want to enjoy life by being in tune. Whether we are aware of it or not, I believe that we all are part of a whole being, which is 'The Creation'. Understand?"

Totally blotting him out, I nod. It's the easiest thing to do when you're high. Just nod.

"Now, you and I have a separate spiritual burden that goes beyond synchronicity. But I can see that you don't care about spiritual burdens right now, because you don't want me to interrupt your high. Yep. I understand, Danny. Believe me, I do. Pot was my first love too."

That part I heard. He creaks down on the bench. He drops his chin on the palm of his hand, and grins at me. It's obvious he wants me to ask him about his romance with the bong, so he and I can relate. Like he thinks the two of us have a connection because we have this unique thing in common. What an idiot. All kids are in love with getting high. I'm just like everyone else from my high school. It's more unusual for a kid to not try it. In fact, compared with a lot of my friends, I was late when I first started. I was fourteen.

Captain drums his fingers against his cheek, waiting to see if I'll bite. He and I do not share some kind of special connection because of pot, and I don't want him to try to buddy up with me about it. He's just looking for any reason to go on and on some more about his whacked-out delusions about synchronicity.

Then again, we really could get more druggies and murderers in here. I hadn't even thought of it until he brought it up about an hour ago. It doesn't take much imagination to see how this night could get much, much worse for me. Captain smells bad, grosses me out, and lives in cuckoo town, but I'll need him on my side. I can tell he wants to be my friend. He could be the difference that gets me out of this hell hole in one piece: my bodyguard. He wants to talk with me about pot? Fine. I'd sure as hell rather talk about weed than hear about hidden cameras.

So, okay, I'll bite. I'm making a crazy friend in jail. "You smoke?"

10:57 PM: Brightening, he lifts his head. "Not anymore. It's too boring now. Now it's crack. After pot, I went to cocaine. And it's always been cocaine. When I'm not locked up, it's the first thing I do every day...which, by the way, is just as valid as everyone else's cup of coffee. It's my bell ringer."

"Oh." Let him burn through his energy. He can't go all night.

"Yeah. My camp has an amazing view of the freeway, which is right below. I'm suspended sixty feet high in the air, like a trapeze artist without a swing, with nothing but a pillar separating me from a free-fall to certain death. But that's life in the fast lane. I'm right above the main artery of the I-5 that heads both north and south. It's actually kind of peaceful. There's the headlights, the tail lights, glowing red through the grey rain. I have to sit or lie down because I've only got about three feet above me. I lean on one elbow and take a hit from my other arm. Danny, that first hit of the day, my bell ringer, is what I live for. You ever try crack?"

"Uh, no."

Excited, he edges toward me. I lean back, holding my knees to my chest. His eyes shining, he croons, "It is instant euphoria. I feel like I've got a million bucks and not a care in the world. I'm enjoying the first rush and I'm happy because I know I have more. I'm alive and it's wonderful! Billions of people lived and now they're dead, but I'm alive! It's a wonderful thing, a phenomenal thing I'm here on this earth. It feels so good just to revel in this thought. It is this feeling that keeps me coming back again and again and forever. The best feeling of all lasts fives minutes. You hear of Freud?"

"Yes."

"He wrote a paper I read which explains how the drug is still working in the body. So it's best to wait fifteen minutes after the first five minute rush and then do another hit — otherwise it's a waste of the crack. It's like drinking fine wine after you're already drunk; you can't taste the difference anymore. So the first hit is the best and then I spend the rest of the day chasing it."

I yawn. Captain chuckles, "Sorry, we were talking about pot." He taps my arm. "I remember when it was pot. It was great for me when I was on a budget. It was so cheap. A joint could get a whole bunch of people stoned. One hit off a joint and I was high for hours. That was fifty cents. I could get a whole ounce for ten bucks. It's your cost-effectiveness of mind altering substances. Yeah, I thought I would smoke pot every day for the rest of my life."

"Really."

"Danny, I thought I'd never live without marijuana. I loved the happy way pot made me feel, don't you? But don't incriminate yourself! Ha ha!"

I nod.

"There ya go, Danny! Yeah, it was fun to get high. It was a relief from stress. It expanded my creativity. It was my enjoyment and entertainment. I only took it when I had time off and when I was with my friends. I'd have small hits. I always kept it on me so I could do just a small toke. It only took a small amount to make me see the beauty of life. There weren't really that many times in my life where I got totally stoned. You know one of the things I liked best about pot?"

"What?"

"That the most valuable part of it is a horny female. You know this, right? You have to sort the stems from the seeds, right? The female plant produces the resin to..."

"Yes, I know. Attract the pollen from the male plant. Yeah."

"Right. So the more a female plant wants the pollen, the more she produces resin, so it makes it..."

"More toxic. And toxic equals THC."

"You got it, Danny. The hornier the female, the better it makes you feel."

"Yes, I know. I read about it."

"Then you must also know that, if you want to get a girl horny, you give her some pot. When I was your age, my friends and I didn't want to have to wait until we were really old to have sex!"

Christ, I do not want to talk about sex with this guy. This is creepy as hell. I shift and look away.

"Danny! You haven't figured that out yet? Always have something to loosen up the ladies."

Oh my God.

"If I ever want to have sex with a woman I just give her what she wants. It will be easy and it will be friendly. I don't drink, but I would happily buy a bottle of wine to get a woman to hang out with me. This is why all the drug dealers have women hanging around them. They've got the *Social Lubricant.* That's what my old girlfriend used to call it: a Social Lubricant. See, without the drugs we wouldn't have a reason to get together. You can't just walk up to a woman and tell her you want to talk to her. But you can walk up to a woman ask her if she wants to get high. See? Proving my point again, Your Honor, the most valuable part about pot is a horny female."

My girlfriend — ex-girlfriend — was definitely someone who liked fooling around when she was high. No way am I gonna say anything to Captain about her. He might dig for details and I'd rather puke. But I made sure I always had something on me so I'd be ready whenever she was ready. Anything to be next to her Pulse jeans, her honey shampooed hair and dirty, smoky laugh.

She would hold my hand in the hallway so everyone could see she was my girlfriend. She'd take our intertwined hands and put them behind her, at the small of her back. With her strawberry-blonde Farrah Fawcett hair billowing at my shoulder, she'd say, "Hey."

I'd look down at her green eyes shining at me.

"Come here." She'd pull on the collar of my shirt and kiss me right in front of everyone. And then she'd swipe on more lip gloss. That used to make me crazy. I could barely get through fifth and sixth periods waiting to kiss her again. Then we'd go to one of our cars, get high, and mess around.

One night, we were making out in the station wagon at a park, a couple miles from my house. We weren't having sex or anything but I think the windows were steamy. The Who was blasting. A cop knocked on my window, and we had to get out so he could search the car. We stood there in the cold, foggy night, our sneakers wet from the dew. He opened up the glove compartment and a baggie of pot fell out. He said he thought he smelled that. He wrote us up a couple of tickets and then he asked if I was okay to drive. I said yes and they drove away. I got behind the wheel and backed right into a muddy ditch.

Technically, this didn't go on our records because we were minors. They brought us before a review board and we were both given community service. It wasn't all that much, really. Getting high with my girlfriend in exchange for ten hours of pulling weeds for the city? I'll make that deal any day. Sure.

The shitty part is Lynette's parents made us break up and banned her from seeing me ever again. She avoided me in the hallway, wouldn't look at me, and sat at a different table in the cafeteria.

But I still see her eyes; I feel her curls in my fingers and her soft lips on my face.

"Come here."

My chest is weighted with heavy stones. I want to roll up in a ball and let the heaviness pull me under the cement floor and make me disappear.

11:10 PM: Captain wistfully gloats, "Yeah, pot works like magic with the opposite sex. They'll do things they wouldn't do otherwise."

No more girl talk. I can't stand it. I motion to the ceiling and say, "How do you know there's someone listening to us?"

"Oh hundreds of reasons, but for right now, I'll just tell you a joke." Captain nods his head toward the guard's station. "I'm so poor I eat the boogers of cocaine addicts."

Beefcake laughs. Okay, so the guard's listening to us. This has nothing to do with The Others. I ask, "I mean, who else? You know, The Others. The ones you say I don't know about?"

He looks at the clock. "What time is it, Danny? You must first tell me the time."

"I checked already. Ten after eleven?"

Captain sighs with disgust. "Didn't anyone teach you how to tell time?" He motions to the clock. "It's not ten after eleven. It's 11:11!"

11:11 PM: It just clicked over. Who gives a shit about one minute?

"That's four ones. There is no other repetition of four numbers of anything when it comes to telling time."

"Oh, right."

"So you should pay attention, Danny. The spirits want you to know something."

"Again?"

"Yes, again! Now is the perfect time. Do you want me to tell you?"

"Uhhh — tell me — what?"

"About The Others! Are you going to let 11:11 pass before it changes? You said you wanted to know!"

"Oh. Oh, right. Yeah. Sure."

He snarls, "'Oh, right, yeah, sure?' Jesus! Like, 'Why not? Whatever? It's no big deal'? Like what I have to say is just made up? That's bullshit, Danny! I've lived a lifetime — day in and day out — with this crown of thorns. You toss out — very sarcastically — that you would do me the favor and kill a little time by hearing about the illicit underworld of our government and my mortal obligation as John the Baptist! All of which you mistakenly think has nothing to do with your privileged, rich ass, self! But it does!"

"Captain, I…"

"It's 11:13 now. You ruined it. Go fuck off."

There's that baby rodent feeling on the back of my neck again. Where's it coming from? I twist to look behind me, then under the bench. Nothing. I know I shouldn't care what a mentally ill person thinks about me, but I can't stand it when Captain tries to make me a part of his crazy-ass story.

11:31 PM: Timing is everything in life. When the parents are mad, I've learned it's best to wait until they stop stomping around before I get to work on them. Angry parents require serious buttering up before I slip and slide out of the consequences. I like to give them a special technique I've developed. It's called the *I Am Still the Son You Know and Love Charm Offensive*. It's a multi-step process.

First, I approach the parent who is no longer hot, but merely simmering. I make my sweetest face. It consists of my most charming smile, my widest eyes, and a sideways tilt of my head. I don't plead for forgiveness or prove how unreasonable the punishment is. No. With youthful sincerity, I ask for his or her advice. This is because the greatest compliment you can give someone is to ask for their help.

I dish up something that shows my generosity as a loving member of our family unit. For example, I'll ask my mom what I should get my sisters for Christmas, or how much sugar I'd need to make the blackberry pie I'm baking for that night's dessert. This really works with them, especially my mom. It makes them feel like even though parenting has its tough moments, it's all been worth it. After I've graciously accepted his or her wise instruction, I mention that my friends are getting together after dinner to study (party), and ask if maybe I could have the car keys. Bingo! It works every time. My consequence is almost always lessened, and once or twice, it's even been entirely forgotten.

Since Captain went completely off the rails with his John the Baptist crown-of-thorns tirade, I figured I'd let him cool his jets before I put my charm offensive in motion. Only thing is, he's been pacing the cell nonstop over the last fifteen minutes. I've even had to tuck my feet under so he won't step on me. Obviously, he wants me to know he's still mad.

Don't want him whipping up any additional anger, so I just get to work on him. I widen my eyes, scratch my head, and act like I didn't do anything that pissed him off. "Captain, uh…could you help me with something?"

"NO!" He keeps pacing. Suddenly, he stops and shouts, "What!?"

"I need a bed roll and a blanket." I tilt my head, widen my eyes. "I want to earn Happy Time, so I want to be sure I say the exact right thing on the kite."

"A kite." He's got a new thought. "Yeah. That's it. A kite. Good idea, smart ass."

Captain marches over and snatches the paper and pencils out of the box. He flings the paper in my direction and then shoves me a pencil. I try to take it from him but he won't let go of it: he's demanding my attention first. "No way am I letting this one go. No way. No way in hell. This time, I'm getting something." Having successfully made his point, he finally lets me take the pencil. Watching him carefully, I pick up the paper.

"So, Captain, what should I say?"

He turns and slams his paper against the wall and scribbles. "Don't bug me. I'm concentrating."

I recite, "Please give me a…"

"No, no, no, Danny. Come on!" He drops his kite and pencil at his sides in exasperation. "Don't just say you want a bed roll. Make it entertaining for them. Give them something to talk about with the wife when they get home. Remember? They're stuck down here in this drab place. They need something fun. Come up with something that complements my booger joke."

Bingo! He's not mad at me anymore. He's easier to steer than my parents.

11:54 PM: Complement a booger joke? As Captain continues to scrawl on his paper, I smirk to myself about how the real joke is on me. I always saw myself inside a jail cell. But I was supposed to be the lawyer! The hero-lawyer defending my client from the great injustices of the world.

Two seemingly contradictory things inspired me to be a lawyer: *High Times* magazine and a TV show called *Perry Mason*. The first time I saw *High Times* I was at a head shop in Pike Place Market. I was drawn inside by their marijuana posters in the window.

The store sells Grateful Dead shirts, rolling papers, stash boxes (that look like a can of Coke to hide drugs in plain sight), and *High Times* magazine. I'll never forget when I first saw the magazine. It was amazing for me to discover there was a life, a whole publication, around pot. *High Times* started as a quarterly issue and recently became monthly. I have every single issue from its first two years.

High Times gives information on how to get pot and how to use it. I know how much to pay for weed because the magazine prints prices charged for Mexican, Thai stick, Madanuska Valley Thunderfuck, etc. It also gives the varying prices around the country. There are articles that explain the difference between organic drugs (peyote) and synthetic ones (LSD).

It's the *Rolling Stone* of the drug lifestyle. The articles about women are always about the hot ones or movie stars. It shows how men should have a little black book full of the phone numbers of waitresses and stewardesses. *High Times* is the inspiration for me to fight to legalize marijuana once I'm practicing law. And when I do become an attorney, I'm going to be just like Perry Mason.

Perry Mason had the cool factor. He had Paul Drake, a private investigator, who went out and found things out for him. He had a secretary that made phone calls for him. They never showed him in casual clothes, he was always in a sharp suit. Perry Mason wasn't married. He was married to the cause of justice. They never showed him dating, but probably all the women loved him. Not only would he get his client off but he would find out who really did it. He was rich but he never talked about money. You never saw him pumping gas, giving Christmas bonuses, or arguing with Paul Drake about his billing rate.

Perry Mason and *High Times* don't contradict each other. They complement each other. Imagine Perry Mason out solving the great injustices of the world (like legalizing marijuana), and celebrating his victory by getting high with a beautiful woman from his little black book. That's going to be me.

Except I never thought I would be the victim of the great injustice who wishes he could hire Perry Mason. A victim unjustly persecuted by being locked up with a hysterical cellmate whose mouth should be a muzzled shut after buckling him down in a straightjacket.

I've made sure I've done almost everything right in my life so I can become a lawyer. Up until tonight, my parents thought I did almost everything right too. But they might feel the need to keep punishing me somehow. My grades were good and I'm moving into the dorms in a couple weeks, but they might decide they should ground me until I leave. While I'm still at home, my charm offensive will have to be *I Am the Son Who Learned His Lesson by Going to Jail and Is Now Thankfully Back On Track.*

Captain juts his papers right under my nose. "Here. Sign it." He looks proud, like this is the end of the trimester and he's handing in a written exam.

"Why are you giving it to me?"

"Your word has to be worth something. Otherwise, they wouldn't have put you here."

"I don't understand. I have to sign your kite?"

"Take it."

I take it and look at what he's written. It's impossible to read: it's a bunch of illegible, tiny, spider-scratch words filling both sides of the paper. "What's it say?"

"It guarantees me my freedom. I deserve my fair share."

"I don't understand. How does my signature…?"

He leans in and spits in my face. "READ IT!! CAREFULLY! THEN SIGN IT! IT'S A CONTRACT, YOU MOUTHY LITTLE SHIT!"

Whoa. And just like that, he's spun out again. I wipe his disgusting, gooey spittle off my face. God. What's he going to infect me with? At least when I get my parents to calm down, they don't blow their lids all over again like this clown.

I'm not arguing with a crazy person. I've watched enough *Perry Mason* to know that a signature of a fake name on a scrap piece of paper from a lunatic cellmate isn't going to hold much weight in a court of law.

I sign it. To pretend I defer and to regain control of him.

His whole arm shaking, he points to the slot in the wall next to the box. "In the slot. Make it official. It will go to the guard. It will be from you. I'm not saying anything — nothing — until you deposit it! Go!"

Scrambling out of my corner, I insert the papers into the slot and put the pencil back in the box. Officer Beef gives the kites and me a passing glance, but only a glance.

"Hurry up!" Looking at the clock, Captain claps his hands in succession. "Let's get started!"

11:58 PM: Started on what?

"It's almost midnight!" Captain commands, "We have to start NOW!"

When I wrote on my kite, I didn't ask for a stupid bedroll. On the off-chance Officer Beef will read it before the morning, and on the even smaller chance he'll feel sorry for me, what I actually wrote was:

"PLEASE PLEASE MAKE SURE HE DOESN'T HURT ME — HE'S CRAZY!"

Captain snaps his fingers under my nose. "Another kite! Get another kite! Hurry up!"

Holy Christ. What did I agree to? I get a new kite. He points to the bench. I veer past him and sit on it. "Okay, okay. It's not midnight yet." The bench is still warm from him sleeping on it. Gross.

"Quit whining! Get in your place NOW! Don't fuck this one up!" He points to the clock. "Fifty-six…" He freezes.

11:59:57: We both watch.

11:59:58: The clock.

11:59:59: Tick.

12:00 AM: "It's midnight!" He jumps like he's won the lottery. "Danny! You know what this means?!"

"It means it's midnight?"

"No, Danny! No!" Elated, Captain grips my shoulders. "Look! The two hands are meeting as one. Like you and me!"

"Yeah?" I wrench away from him by stretching to look at the clock.

He points his arms straight up over his head, the way the hands on the clock look when it's midnight. "They are pointed toward the heavens! PM has turned to AM! When it turns this way again it will be high noon!" He dances like he's trying to fly. "All the magical, special things happen at the stroke of midnight! The animals talk, the carriage turns into a pumpkin! I can do whatever I want! This will happen tonight!"

He raises his fists in victory, then dances in a circle like Rocky Balboa. He shakes his shoulders, but then he slows to a stop. His face falls. It seems like he's listening to someone I can't hear.

He turns and stalks toward me. His nostrils flare. His voice is heavy. "Midnight means I have the extra force behind me. I have the power. And I'm changing the direction of things."

He keeps doing this — switching from light to dark. He does it so fast I don't know he's switched until he's there already. And — here's the real problem — he blames me for whatever he's mad about.

I have no clue what's going on in his crazy brain. But I must steer him back to happy-land. I say, "Midnight. That's great! You're going to change the direction!"

"Now! I mean right now!"

"Uhh…Yes, great! That's great! Right now."

But he's getting more frustrated. "I'm getting paid! This is the time! You get it? Do you understand?"

"Yes! Yes, I understand perfectly."

"No, you don't get it!'"

"I do, Captain, it's changing. Right now!"

"You don't see! You don't appreciate who I am!" He widens his eyes. He bends toward me. I guess so he can give me a better view of the red veins spread like thorns over his yellow eyeballs. "I am John the Baptist."

I mirror him. Widen my eyes, so he sees I'm amazed. "Yes, uh, I do, Captain. I do. I get it. This is pretty amazing."

"Good. Good." He nods and backs away. "Because I've survived everything, Danny! I've lived on locusts! For years! And they've been closing in on me so I've had to take extra precautions. They've been watching my spiritual work a lot closer now. They spied on me from an apartment on The Ave. The Holy Spirit told me. So every time I walked by, I had to duck my head and pull my hood tight around my face. But I refuse to go down. I will not be crushed under their pressure. I am getting paid. Finally. I'm getting paid. For my life! They are not getting my wisdom for free! Not anymore!" He points at me. "And NEITHER ARE YOU!"

I knew it. I knew he'd find a way to be mad at me. "Hey, I told you, remember? I said before, I don't want anything from you!"

"Yes, you do! You asked me about The Others!"

"The what?"

"Danny! THE OTHERS WHO ARE WATCHING US THROUGH HIDDEN CAMERAS!"

"Oh — right." I am so confused. I forgot about The Others. "Look, if you don't want to…"

"But that cost me! I've been shunned! Starved! Cold! Wet! For years! This is my expense, Danny! My human expense! I lived under a freeway overpass! I took my life in my hands every time I left my camp. I crossed a freeway exit every single day, Danny! For years! Do you realize that?"

"Uh, no…'

"No, you don't! Yesterday morning — it's rush hour — cars hydroplane by me going eighty miles an hour. If I'm not on high-octane alert — if I stumble — I'm road kill — like living in a war zone — cars roaring past — blowing wind and rain — I hold onto a light pole in case I need to jerk myself back — in case I get run over — but I see a break in traffic so I get ready…"

He positions himself like he's in the starting line for a race, he continues, "One, two, three…I pump my arms — and race across for my life. But then a BMW careens around the bend!" He measures the distance between him and me. "The driver's face and mine are almost as close as I am to you. His eyes pop out of his head — his mouth says, 'OH!' I scream, 'FUCK' — I hurdle faster!"

Captain pretend-dives in front of me, skimming past my knees. I pull my legs up, and complain, "Hey…"

He crashes into the corner, breathless. "He swerves. I feel the vibration of his car — hot against me — it rocks my torso and scrapes my ankle." Captain brushes his side. "Then another driver splashes water on me —damn it! I'll be cold for hours! Then he fucking honks at me! People honk at me all the time, Danny. Fuckers. Don't give a shit what any of them think. God approves of my life on the edge."

He shakes his fist at the disinterested taillights. His hand slows to a stop at his side. He stands there like he's wet on the side of the freeway. I can almost see his hair blowing as the cars zoom past him. His gaze parks on the floor. Seems like he's recovered from his brush with death so I slowly let my feet back down.

He muffles, "I've almost died thirty times on that stretch of asphalt." He gears his head in my direction. "But I always made it across." His eyes flick wide with fury and high-beam into mine. He screeches, "And I'm still alive!"

Oh, no. Oh, shit. "Captain, uh, I…"

He cuts me off, "And you want the privilege of looking in and sorting through it?"

"I don't actually…"

He accelerates toward me, pointing his hands to his chest. "To find out where exactly my camp is located. Which exact overpass my camp is under? So you can find it. Just like you tried to find out which exact coffee shop is the one where you can find Sage. So you can make a score without giving me my cut? Are you some kind of thief? Or sick voyeur? You want to take my experience and piece through it, examine it, for your own curiosity or edification so you can gain something from me?"

"No, Captain, I…Let's just forget I asked."

"Danny, you do not understand that this is an honor for you! A great honor. But I am not giving it away for free."

"It's okay, Captain. It was a mistake. I didn't know what I was—"

"My life is precious. Not a cheap peep show!"

"We don't have to talk about it!"

"Oh, yes we do! We made the transaction. The kite. Your signature. That's binding. This means I get a huge pay day. A big chunk! To pay me back! So don't mess up my pay day. I mean it, Danny, don't you fuck this up!"

"I won't."

"Because if that's what you're doing…"

"No. I'm not!"

"I won't let you take it from me!" His nose collides with mine. He grabs my shoulders. I'm afraid to move away this time. His lips are revving so tight they're white. If I say the wrong thing, do the wrong thing, he'll run me over.

Very carefully, I promise, "I won't mess it up." He checks me to see if I'm telling the truth. I have no idea what I won't mess up. Frozen, I hold my innocent expression. Swallow. He breathes fast and loud through his nostrils.

He hurls my shoulders back. Speeds away from me.

I steady myself on the bench. Exhale.

12:11 AM: Captain's had his back to me, staring into the guard's window, for several minutes. Beef never bothered to look up at him. Not even when he was crashing into the wall.

It's a huge relief to not have Captain coming at me. It was bad enough when he tapped my arm. But getting in my face? Grabbing my shoulders? Pushing me back? What the hell? Doesn't he see how much stronger I am? Like I said, I do not want to fight him. I don't need any extra trouble from law enforcement. But if it's him or me, I could easily break his twiggy collar bone.

Less than eight hours and I'll be free from this living hell. In less than eight hours, Steve will pick me up in his dad's Mercedes.

Whenever I ride in their car I feel like a rich kid. Before we got our driver's licenses, Steve's dad used to drive us to a freestyle skiing class. I was already stoked about going because it was a class for only expert skiers. But when we pulled up in the Mercedes, all the other skiers would turn to stare at us. Steve and I would step out slowly and we'd carefully take down our equipment. That way, there was more time for all those people in their plain cars to enjoy our Mercedes show. We felt like rock stars.

The only car I'm allowed to drive is our old, blue station wagon. Talk about embarrassing. Other parents help their kids get cool, used cars or pass down their old Honda or something. But I get this beater-dented-mommy-family-car that's the size of a blimp that I have to share with my younger sister who just turned sixteen. The only benefits to that station wagon are it goes fast and there's plenty of room for making out in the front seat, back seat, and the trunk.

My dad drives a Mustang II. It can fit five people if we squish three in the back. Since my mom starting working, she bought a Cutlass Supreme. It can fit five a little more comfortably. But we don't ever need to do that. All four of us kids rarely go somewhere with either one of our parents anymore.

The station wagon is the only car in the family that fits a family of six. That's the car we took when we went to church, to see Grandma, or to see our cousins for Thanksgiving. We took it on ski trips, family vacations, and towing the camper up to the mountains. We'd take our dog and cats with us in the car. When we'd leave for a long drive, we wouldn't pull out of the driveway until our dad led us all in a family prayer for our safe return.

Now the station wagon is the teenagers' car. It's the car the parents don't care about anymore.

In the morning, I will not be picked up from jail in a Mustang II or a Cutlass Supreme. I begged and pleaded with Steve to get himself out of bed and come get me. He will pull up in the Mercedes like he's my private chauffeur. He'll push open the passenger side door and a haze of smoke will waft out and fill my senses. He'll smile and welcome me inside by handing me a lit joint. Then we'll drive away and with each lungful of bliss I'll blow this nightmare, and Captain, out of my brain.

Steve's dad won't care if the Mercedes comes back smelling like pot because he smokes too. Steve's older brother was the one who got Steve into it and Steve was the one who got me high for the first time. We were night skiing.

I remember I sliced the edge of my skis up an icy hill past a sign that read: DANGER — KEEP OUT. We followed Steve into a forest where the other night skiers couldn't see us. Steve whispered to me, "Dibs on Donna."

"Which one's Donna?"

"The blonde."

Was this a double date? The three of them had been chatting constantly since the time we met them in the lodge about an hour before. I hadn't ever been on a date or anything. Those girls were drawn to Steve like a magnet. He was pretty laid back about it because he was used to girls fawning all over him.

I remember turning around to look at the girls because I wanted to see if they noticed me. They hadn't. The other reason was my nose was dripping from the cold and I ran out of tissues, so I had to wipe the snot off my shoulder without being obvious about it.

Through the branches, I saw the lights glowing on the slope. They looked like birthday candles going down the mountain. As we pushed off and skied deeper into the woods, it was like someone had blown out the candles and everything became dark.

The girls probably thought I was a loser because I didn't say anything. But I figured I'd make up for it when we left the off-limits trail. I planned to show off for them on the moguls with hot-dogger skiing, casual flips and a 360.

When we arrived in a clearing, Steve shifted his skis around to face us. I still couldn't think of anything clever to say, so I used my ski glove to dab at my water faucet nose. It was like they spoke a different language from me. It was the same feeling I got when I'd walk past the popular kids' table at school, like I was outside their circle.

Then he took it out. It was the first time I had ever seen a joint up close before. It was inside a baggie: stuffed in his pocket along with mints, a few bucks, wadded up tissues, and a lighter.

I was a little curious about it, but I wasn't going out looking for it or anything. Was he going to share it with us? Did he expect me to try it? I didn't even know if I wanted to. Right then? On an off-limits trail? But I didn't want to look stupid if I didn't take a hit. I worried about doing it wrong and if the girls would laugh at me or not. They couldn't take their eyes off Steve as he stuck the joint between his lips.

He lit up without even saying anything about it. He didn't ask if the girls wanted to or not. He just did it. He acted like we were all okay with it. He was right. Like it was the same thing as handing me a mint, he passed the joint to me.

I thought about the people at church and how they wouldn't approve.

Then I saw the girls smiling at me. This was the first time they actually saw me. They were waiting for me to hurry up and take a hit so they could take a turn. The snow sprinkled their feathered hair and eyelashes like sugar on doughnuts. I would have gone for either of them but I could tell both of them put dibs on Steve.

As I looked at the joint Steve was holding out for me, I figured this must be what you do with a girl you like. No one had told me how to go on a date or hang around a girl. I didn't know when to hold hands, or what to talk about. I didn't know when the right time was to kiss a girl. Smoking a joint seemed like as good an idea as any other. In fact, on that maybe-double date, it was obvious smoking pot would help me achieve something.

I figured I had my life planned out. I knew if I tried a little pot, there would be no way it would get in the way of my goals. I may have forgotten my tissues, but I didn't forget my list of goals. It was in my ski jacket.

Then I realized it had been a long time since we'd been to church.

I took the joint. I sucked it in the way Steve did. It felt like breathing in smoke from a campfire, but more velvety than scratchy. Copying Steve, I held it in my lungs. Steve nodded for me to pass the joint to not-Donna, so I did. When I saw Steve exhale, I exhaled too.

I didn't feel anything.

But I had something to do with my hands. Passing a joint made me feel like I spoke their language, like I had something to talk about. Holding the joint, and sucking in the incense-like smoke, made me feel like I didn't have to worry if I wasn't as cool as Steve or I had boogers on my jacket. As the joint got passed around, we huddled in closer.

I was in their circle.

12:43 AM: I think Captain forgot I'm here. Christ, I hope so. I'm trying to be really still and quiet so I don't break his trance.

Every couple minutes Captain would mumble. He'd scratch his scalp with his knuckles that are lined with deep, blackened grooves. Then he'd examine his long, thick nails to inspect what he picked out of his head. He did this a few times. Each morsel was like a new discovery for him.

I'll be coming down soon. How will I tolerate Captain? I can't stand it when I need a buzz but can't get it. A month ago, I ran out of pot while I was working in Alaska and I thought I would completely lose my mind.

It was seven days in fishery hell without any pot whatsoever. Seven days since I smoked the very last remnant of what I had brought with me. Just one little hit could have gotten me through a few hours. Then a booster hit for another few and, hell, I could have hacked the heads off salmon all day long.

When I applied for the job in Alaska I assumed it would be like every other job I've ever had, except way more money. I had jobs as a busboy, a dishwasher. I sold blackberries door to door, had a paper route. It's not like I didn't know how to work. But nothing could have prepared me for the heavy, grueling labor of the fishing boats and canneries. All I wanted to do was escape. But it was way too complicated getting in and out of that place. I flew from Seattle to Alaska and then took a seaplane to Podunk, Nowhere. I was stuck for the duration.

It was all Joss's fault. He went up a couple weeks ahead of me so he should have warned me how bleak it was there. Nothing was funny. The world was hateful. Life wasn't worth living. It was all I could do to not yell at everybody. We did horrible things: we'd throw live crabs into a mattress-sized basket of hot brine. The crabs would snatch the bars with their little claws. We knew when they died because their claws would release. It was a shit show. I was relieved at least not to have to hear them scream.

"FINISH UNLOADING!" the fisherman hollered at me. He waved Joss over to go talk to him. I thought he was going to give Joss crap for not moving his ass fast enough.

I squatted down and plunged my hands into the ice. I dug for the scaly, frozen fish and pitched it. I was a living contradiction of hot and cold — ice chipped on my burning, sweating face and melted down my neck. Joss and I had been doing this on and off for ten hours that day. For the previous six hours my legs had been shaking uncontrollably and I couldn't feel my hands anymore.

There were only two girls working at the cannery and I heard they cried themselves to sleep every night. There was nothing to do other than work. I mean nothing. It was like nature and civilization went to war for this place, but nature won with a vengeance. No entertainment. No police. No hospital. No grocery store, just a convenience store that was ripping everybody off for a loaf of bread and bologna. And milk? Forget it. It was way too expensive. Joss and I were drinking powdered milk in our hot cereal, which was one of our two menu choices every single fucking shitty meal.

The memory of getting high overwhelmed my every waking thought. How the smoke would fill my lungs and I'd hold it, hold it. Exhale. Soon I would have the careless feeling of wafting up and over life's challenges. One tiny toke and I wouldn't have hated Alaska or my job. And I wouldn't have been pissed off at Joss for not saying one single thing in his letters about how cold and wet and depressed I was going to be every minute of every hour of every day.

It was dangerous up there too. They used saw blades. And there wasn't even a doctor! They had to airlift out a couple guys who were gushing blood.

There were two liquor stores. Some guys bought us some beer, but, honestly, having a drink was nothing compared to getting high. Nothing. One hit before bedtime would have helped me sleep in my dirty, stained, lumpy bunk. It felt like there was no way I could make it.

As I unloaded the last ugly salmon I ever wanted to see, Joss walked over to me, grinning from ear to ear, carrying a halibut. This was salmon season. What was he doing with that?

"Oh, you are going to be so happy."

"Why?"

"The fisherman gave it to us. He can't use it."

"Are you serious?" My mouth was watering. It had been three weeks since I ate anything other than cereal and bologna sandwiches.

"And check this out..." Joss lifted the fish. Nestled underneath it was a little sandwich baggie of pot.

Oh. My. God. I was speechless.

Joss said with great reverence and joy, "It's Madanuska Valley Thunderfuck."

There are some pots that are legendary. I had heard about Madanuska Valley Thunderfuck for years. Two hours later, I saw how it had righteously earned its reputation. Joss and I sat on our bunks, deliriously happy. We could not stop smiling.

There is nothing as satisfying as having an itch you can scratch.

To have had my cravings satisfied with Madanuska Valley was like feeling the sunshine on my face after weeks of unrelenting rain. But it ruined every other kind of weed for me in the world because it was the perfect feeling of total bliss. It was like being in love for the first time.

12:59 AM: Like he suddenly realized something, Captain sharply turns around. His hair fans out. Tangled strands stick to the stubble on his face. He stares at me.

Oh, Christ. What now?

He looks confused. Good. Confused is good. It's too hard to handle him when he's mad. His massive Adam's apple rolls up and down as he looks around the cell. "Danny." It's almost a question.

I clear my throat, "Yeah?"

"Where…where were we? I lost my focus."

"Let me think." Good. I'm setting the course. "I know! You were going to tell me another joke."

Captain smacks his hands to his ears. He sighs heavily. I guess he didn't fall for it. He moans, "*Ohnnnn…*" With exaggerated exhaustion, he drags his claws down his face, pulling his outer eye lids. His face gargoyles into a Halloween mask. "Jokes? Are you fuuuucking kidding me!?"

"Come on, Captain, your jokes are funny."

"Okay. Danny. Shut up. Okay?" He puts his hands together in prayer. "Just shut up for one damn minute. Your ignorance is deafening." He opens his hands. "Are you really this stupid? I'm trying to tell you things that will help you. You act like you don't understand that you really fucking need to know what I'm going to tell you."

"I've wanted to ask you some more about THC."

His face quivers, "You asshole! I said shut up! God! Teenagers!" He closes his eyes for a moment. Trying to muster up some patience, he slowly opens them. "Are you listening now?"

"Uh. Yes."

"To me?"

"Yes."

Like he's talking to a toddler who has hearing problems, Captain enunciates, "You see, Danny, this has been the process for centuries. In biblical times, kings used to pay to have people interpret their dreams or read their fortunes. A king would seek out the prophet — usually a poor person — who would have the superior knowledge the king would want. Yes? *Comprende?*"

"Yes."

He's back. Full speed again. "That's why there are microphones and cameras in here. It's the same thing going on in here, except the kings paid their philosophers and sages a portion of their wealth. They gave them one-twelfth of their food and gold. With the Greeks; the wealthy would hire a tutor to teach their children one on one. Like Merlin taught Arthur. That's why you're alone in this cell with me. Now do you understand, you imbecile? So I can teach you and so they can have it for the record to watch over and over and so they can learn from it. But I'm only talking now because, like I said, now I'm getting paid for it. Damn it. I'm getting my freedom! So, are you ready to sit still and shut up? And take notes?"

"So…you want me to take notes?"

"Are you deaf?"

"No. No."

"Then quit interrupting with stupid questions."

"Okay, but…" I don't know what to say that won't set him off. "I'm, I'm ready."

He waits until my eyes are on him. "The secret to surviving tough times is to handle your wolves. We all have two wolves inside us that are at constant battle. One wolf is evil: full of anger, jealousy, sorrow, regret, false pride. The other wolf is good. It's joy, love, serenity, hope. Tell me, Danny, which wolf do you think wins the battle?"

"The good one?"

"The one you feed." He gets too far into my personal space again, shedding his loosened flecks of dandruff onto my lap. "The one you feed."

He retreats and paces slowly. When he turns his back, I flick his flakes off me.

"So, in each day, you need to be the best person you can be at that moment. Don't worry about tomorrow or seven days from now. It's all about this one day and getting the most you can out of that day. And there are opportunities everywhere for you to do that. There are people all over that you can meet and make their lives better. Why aren't you writing that down?

You're supposed to be taking notes. Write that down!" I do. "At any moment the burning bush could come up and talk to you. The question is: will you choose to stop and listen or will you go on your way to get drugs?"

God. I wish I didn't make friends with him. I should have ignored him.

"Eye contact, Danny. Look at me. I'm talking to you."

1:10 AM: "You'll come upon weird situations and people. The important thing is to not get flustered. For example, you'll meet people who appear to be interested in you. Odd. Why are they so interested? Because they have an ulterior motive. Know this and keep your cool. There's nothing to be done about it. Just accept it. This person could be a messenger from the spirit world — and you can tell if they are because there will be a glow around him or her — and they'll be very calm. A messenger from heaven is always unafraid. The other possibility is the person is from the Central Intelligence Agency."

"What?" I don't want to stop him and drag this out any longer than I have to, but now I actually do want to know what the hell he's thinking.

He squares himself with me. "The CIA. That's who's watching us, Danny. All the time and in all kinds of ways. It's the CIA, and all their rich friends. They are The Others. That is the answer to the question you asked me at 11:10. And then at 11:11 when you fucked up the situation so irreparably, I had to wait for a better time, which turned out to be right now at 1:11 AM. A time that tells us — you, most importantly — to pay attention."

1:11 AM: "So, how do you know it's the CIA?"

"Look, this isn't the first time the CIA has had me conduct an experiment in jail. NASA wanted to see how a group of Alpha Males would get along in a small space together. You see, they were planning a space flight to Mars. So they put a whole crowd of angry motherfuckers all in one tiny holding cell with me. It was too tight. Things were getting claustrophobic and tempers were flaring. But I knew what was happening. I knew we were being observed. So, I calmly explained to everyone what was really going on with NASA and the CIA. Then they were cool and we all got along. For eighteen straight hours together, without room for anyone to lie down. Because of me. Because of me, NASA took a space ship full of Alpha Males to Mars. So obviously tonight, the CIA has given me another difficult assignment." He raises his eyebrows at me, "Because they know I can handle it. Handle you."

"And why are they watching us?"

"Pay attention! I told you this already! We're Chosen people! Jesus, Danny! We've got less than seven hours. After that, you're on your own and you're going to wish you could ask me questions! And wish you had written down every single one of my words! I've got a lot of material to go over with you and you're making me circle back and review what I just told you? Don't throw me off my train of thought again! Are you fucking insane?!"

"Sorry."

"There's someone in a limousine right now waiting for a tape of you and me to be delivered to him. So he — and his rich friends — can entertain themselves by watching us and studying us. In fact, the only place I knew where I could truly hide from them was in my camp. I could light my candles, play with my cards, and connect with the spirits — and they never found me, they were never able to record my spiritual work. That's why I kept my camp all this time, even though it was so dangerous to get in and out of there. They will go to extremes to watch the Chosen. Our raw footage. Someone's life is another person's short story they watch. Read. They made a deal with the police to get their hands on our time here tonight and so they can eat up every last crumb of my words of wisdom."

"Oh, now I understand."

Weird. "Word of Wisdom" is something they say in the church we used to go to. It's called The Church of Jesus Christ of Latter-day Saints. Everyone calls us *Mormons*. I haven't heard anyone talk about the "Word of Wisdom" since we stopped going there about four years ago. Even though we don't go anymore, I still consider myself a Mormon. When I get married, I'll have my ceremony in a Mormon church.

He says, "I made it harder for the CIA to watch me by constantly moving and walking around."

I ask, "How do you know you're Chosen?" That's another thing they used to tell us in church; that the Mormons are Chosen people.

"Hard evidence, Danny. I have evidence from The Freedom of Information Act. But that's secondary. Later, later. First, you should understand one primary fact. The reason I know I'm Chosen is the angels talk to me. They talk to me every day in all kind of ways that I must detect, and must use my exquisite gifts to understand what they're telling me. We're in contact all the time."

What exquisite horseshit. I nod. "Really?"

"Angels only talk to people who are pure. I am a prophet. I'm special. So God talks to me. And that's why the CIA's after me — and now you."

There's that rodent feeling scratching across the back of my neck. I shrug it away.

He pontificates, "I am the center of the universe with the Holy Spirit giving me messages. The CIA wants to know how I'm getting their messages and how it is that I am the center of all this spiritual tension. And I know I'm living right because God is still communicating with me. That's why I've been living this extraordinary life: to receive His holy messages. No messages from heaven if you're not living right. Write that down."

"No messages from heaven…"

"In fact, my very own ambassadors from heaven would check on me. They are God's angels on earth who regularly came by to visit my camp. Their names are Tracer and Greyshift. I loved watching the blue lights which would trace after them. Their visits were my confirmation I was important and was being cared for from above."

I can't help but ask, "Did they have to cross the freeway too?"

"I don't know. They're rats."

1:23 AM: "I see you watching the clock, Danny. You're always checking the time. You like numbers too, don't you?"

"I dunno. I like to know what time it is."

"I set my life by it. That way, I make the best choices and usually avoid dangerous mistakes — which I didn't do this morning. But — 1:23 AM? That's a fantastic time. Those are sequential numbers: 1-2-3! That's a good indication we're moving in the right direction, besides the twenty-three element — which I'll go into later. So, get up! Let's get some more kites!" He pushes me toward the pencil holder "Now, my underground drug business is a tightrope between life and death, Danny. Life and death."

I take a couple kites. He snaps his fingers. "Just take all of them. Come on, come on."

What the hell does John the Baptist expect me to write? Clutching my school supplies, I sit back down on the warm bench. As long as he's not freaking out on me, I'll just let

Captain Fantastic keep on talking about rat ambassadors and any other hallucination he pulls out of his pickled brain. I was wrong thinking he couldn't talk all night. It's the opposite. He's in the spotlight and feeding on it.

Careful to act obedient and interested, I pretend to take notes.

1:47 AM: "To stay in contact with the spirit world I needed a regular supply of drugs. So the most important person in my life was my dealer, White. White shirt, white bandana, white Trans Am. Get it?"

"I think so."

"Details are very important, Danny, especially when we're talking about my supplier. So I'll tell you, step by step, what went down yesterday. As usual, I called her from The Red Hen. There's an entry area where not even the bartender can see me. He was busy, anyway, with his regular 8:00 AM potatoes throwing their pensions away on pull tabs. I pumped a quarter into the pay phone and called White. We agreed to meet in thirty minutes. Thirty is a good number. I had my twenty bucks saved from the deals I made the day before so I could score first thing in the morning. I hung up. I always loved the sound of the quarter clanking through that black box because it meant a deal was in the works. Next to the payphone, I found a packet of salted crackers and a receipt. Took both of them and went back outside. The receipt had several numbers on it, a pattern…three ones. And as you know, three of any number is a warning."

Captain whips a pencil from the holder and gashes 111 on the wall. He points to them. "Angels were warning me, Danny. Must have been a forewarning about the undercover cop who busted me this morning. Anyway, I drew my hood tighter." He tucks his fist under his chin, bows his head, and ogles side to side as he says, "I looked left and right, but didn't see anyone. It was raining, but the thought of satisfying my constant craving added a joy and bounce to my step." He thumps his hand to his heart, exclaiming, "What a feeling — I scored! It was going to happen! See, Danny, I knew I was helping people and living with God's approval so He wanted me to have what I wanted to feel good. I hotfooted around pot holes in time to a Rachmaninoff piece I had stuck in my head all week. I ate one of the crackers but saved the other for Tracer and Greyshift…"

Rachmaninoff is perfect theme music for Captain because it's like the score from an old fashioned horror film. What I would give to be out of here and back in my living room, sitting on our plush couch, watching my mom's hands climbing up and down her grand piano's keyboard, her brow tense with concentration.

Captain hums the tune. Shit. I'll never enjoy listening to Rachmaninoff after tonight because it will always remind me of him.

"At the coffee shop, I scanned the crowd for cops." Captain squints. "One time, White saw a cop car before I did, which almost never happened. She just tore out of there. She didn't come back and didn't answer her phone for a long time until she thought it was safe. That sucked — that really sucked! There's nothing like having the money and not being able to get what you want. Yesterday, when she came around the corner in her Trans Am…I cannot express the relief I felt to see her car — it was indescribable." Captain shakes his head and sighs, "Every single time I saw her car, it was a relief I felt in my whole body. I got in and smelled peanut butter. White's five-year-old kid was in the back seat, strapped into his kid chair. His jacket zipped up to his chin; he clutched his brown sack lunch to his chest. I don't know if he thought I wanted to take it, or what, but he was just staring at me. No one said hello or anything. White pulled out. The windshield wipers were *thunking.*"

Captain mindlessly doodles over the numbers on the wall. "I met White when she was pregnant and I still don't know her kid's name. I wonder what he tells the other kids at school, because he's old enough to be curious about what his mom's doing. He's seen her pick me up several times in his short life. I wonder what she tells him. White started out dealing with her boyfriend. They ended up breaking up and she became a single mom, got on welfare, saved her drug money, and bought her car. She went from riding a bicycle to driving a Trans Am — all on crack money. She doesn't look like a dealer at all; she doesn't wear makeup, she rarely wears jewelry, she just runs around in a white shirt and jeans looking like a welfare mom. White is probably the oldest dealer out there. She's twenty-four."

Smiling, Captain turns back around. "I guess that makes me a senior citizen because I'm forty-eight. There aren't any old dealers on the streets; either they overdose, get killed, or go to prison. That's probably why the people I did business with trusted my judgment so much; I have a lifetime more experience than almost everybody. And I was still on my perch."

He folds his arms then points the pencil at me. "White's a good dealer for several reasons. She's really reliable and, like a good dealer, never dips into her own stash. I think the only thing she ever did was pot. She's the only one who's up at eight o'clock in the morning because of her kid. Most dealers stay up drinking Hennessey and getting stoned until they pass out on someone's couch until fucking noon the next day. See how a mother makes a good dealer?"

"Sounds like it."

"Not only that, she and I always did a regular exchange: her baggie for my twenty. We never had to talk about it. It was the same deal every time. That's another reason I needed her. There's no Better Business Bureau in the drug world. If I couldn't get drugs from her, I would've had to find them from someone else, and maybe that dealer would give me a little less for my money. Or I couldn't rely on him to have it, or to answer his phone, or whatever. And if I was high, I didn't want to have to deal with a whole bunch of new situations. So, as usual, White gave me a baggie with pieces of crack gathered in a corner and held shut with a little twisty. Most people like to get the whole rock but I liked the crumbs and that's why she gave me such a good deal."

Captain writes 33 on the wall. "I always got out of White's car at the same stop sign. Yesterday, the wipers *thunked* thirty-three times. Three is a magical number; therefore, I knew I was having a magical moment. All was right. Everything was perfect in the world. I didn't need insurance. I gave her my most charming smile and politely let her know how nice it was to see her before I slammed the door and ran off to get high."

He puts his pencil nub next to me on the bench. "I wonder if White uses the same baggies for her crack deals as she does for her kid's peanut butter sandwiches."

2:26 AM: "To earn money to buy my own crack, I was a 'pony boy', which is basically a middle man, in drug deals. But I preferred to call myself an *Urban Industrial Leisure Engineer.* So, if you were a rich working stiff and you had a couple hundred dollars to spend on a Friday night to justify your going to work on Monday morning, I could help engineer how you were going to spend it. That was my job. Society has a place for everybody. The world doesn't need another rich stiff; the world needs someone to hook people up with crack. If you're someone with money, you do coke. You see, cocaine is the drug of status and menace. Now, when I was doing deals, I hid my spiritual powers. No contact with the spirit world while I was dealing because I couldn't pay attention to everything all at once…"

Whackjob.

2:37 AM: "All deals worked around a twenty dollar bill. The trick was to find a dealer who would sell me the pot or a piece of crack for fifteen dollars. Then I made five from the dealer, five from the customer. Ten was the minimum amount I needed to get high. I needed about one hit an hour." Captain laughs, "Those dealers! It's like they all come out of high school smoking blunts, selling crack, and packing heat. These kids don't want to work at a fast food restaurant when they can make good money selling a sack of rocks. It's like someone took them aside and told them how to make a living: what the prices are, how to see if someone's a cop and how to change their name. It's standard they all have made up names for themselves. Capone, Diamond, Black, Red, Blue, White, Smoke, Jeda Jay. And, Danny, it is standard not to ever go to their houses. That's a good way to get shot, tapping on their window. The guns. It is fucking dangerous. Only go with an invitation. Why are you making that face?"

"Just…uh…what's a blunt?"

"It's a cigar where you dig out the tobacco and replace it with marijuana."

I'll definitely remember that one.

2:54 AM: "Another danger is when the crack dealers try to get control over a person. If they have a crack addict who's living in a house, they'll come on over and take over a room — or the whole house — like a home invasion. The dealers will keep pumping them with crack and they'll keep on running drug deals in their house all day, all night. They'll trash the place inside and out until someone finally calls the police. If you're in low-income housing you could lose your place to live forever. But look, it's Seattle. Drug addicts need somewhere inside to get high just like everyone else."

Officer Beef is not looking at me. On purpose! It's been like this for hours. He acts like I'm not even here. All he cares about at his drab government job is his submarine sandwich and cookies.

Yes, I got caught smoking pot but I don't deserve this endless blathering. I never thought I'd come across someone who could lecture me longer than my own parents. I'm so tired and wish he would shut the fuck up. If Captain fell asleep I might take a chance and close my eyes…but Captain would much rather talk about himself than sleep. I am truly his captive audience. Seriously, who gives a shit? How can he not know this? I have to stay awake and not let down my guard in case he spins out again.

Beef! Look at me! Read my kite!

3:08 AM: "I always kept an eye out and knew who was on the block. That's what it's called: *on the block*. Repeat, Danny."

I repeat, "On the block."

"I gave myself thirty minutes to get a deal done or I gave my client their money back. Because the customer was always right. If they were looking for drugs on a Saturday night, they didn't want to wait around for a couple hours! So the closer the better." He rubs his hands together. "It was good to spread it around so I maintained relations with a lot of them. I memorized the numbers of twenty dealers so I was never, ever without one."

When Captain first started in on the drug talk, I'll admit it was kind of interesting. But after hours of drugs, drugs, and more drugs, it's boring as hell. Even for me. Doesn't he want anything else out of life? I used to think my parents' lives were boring, but they at least are interested in a lot of different things. They do stuff. Captain's life is all about hustling money to get high. But outside? Outside in Seattle, where it rains practically every day. How can he live like that?

3:21 AM: Three, two, one. Like a musician counting down at the beginning of a song. Interesting, the numbers are going backwards. I wonder: does that mean we're moving in the wrong direction?

"So you understand the connection here, Danny? Angels wouldn't connect with me if I wasn't a trustworthy businessman, right?"

"*Pure*, I think you said."

"Danny! That's an A-plus! You're paying attention!" He offers me a calloused and scratchy hi-five. I do it. I wipe my hand on my pant leg as I adjust my kites. "I stayed pure by not ripping people off. I was about as legit as you could get in an illegal business."

Captain's words and arm keep time to a distant metronome I just now notice. Is the *tick, tick* coming from the guard's station? In time, Captain says, "Purse snatchers go snatching, get high. Then they go out and look for more purses to snatch. I knew a guy who'd jack coins out of a newspaper machine. Some junkies will stand outside a cash machine for eight hours waiting for someone to forget to take their card. Eventually, someone does and they clear out their account. Me? I was fully engaged in my business and used all my mental resources to make it work well."

Tick, tick. Captain's arms bounce and cut the air in time as he clacks on, "One time, it was snowing. I had a client who gave me a hundred dollars to get him some crack. I took his money to find someone to buy from. I couldn't find anyone because of the snow. I was flat broke, Danny. Freezing and hungry. But no one was selling. I could have run off with my client's money but I gave it back. It hurt to do it, but I gave him his money back. The next week he came back and he was my customer for four years. One time, a dealer and a customer offered me money to kill the customer's wife. Of course, I would never do that, Danny. Never. I never stole from anyone or hurt anyone to run my business or to get high. That's why the spirits trust me."

Satisfied with himself, he folds his arms to the *tick*, then continues, "I was so good at my business that, every now and then, I could attract a rich customer with a couple hundred bucks. Then I'd have money and I could get a magazine, cards, candles, all my drugs, and I'd go back to my camp and connect with the spirits. If I gave up drugs, Danny, I also gave up a special tie I had to the spirit world. This connection was something I could never go back on. I couldn't act like I didn't know about the angels who were watching over me."

He points his finger at me and calls out, "Got that?" The *ticks* cut off. Like he shut them off.

4:20 AM: It just happened. I am no longer stoned. Holy shit. The opposite of 4:20 PM. To the minute! Like some sick fuck is playing a prank on me!

My back, neck, and shoulders are burning. I've been scribbling on tiny pieces of paper on my lap for so long the hard bench has permanently deformed my sit bones and flattened my ass. Nothing to rest my back on unless I move to the cold, hard floor.

"Messages from the spirits can be received through various means. Things are connected that don't seem connected at all. A crow will caw. It tells me nature agrees with me. A guy will say something that turns out to be a sign from heaven. See, I also get messages from angels through other people. How? First, I listen. Then I take a word they said and that will be an indicator of the message. For example: the word 'wheel'. Take the first letter: 'w', and last one: 'l'. Which brings you to 'win lost'; which means I no longer have that person on my team. Like the win was actually lost. I won them over and then I lost them. So, how do I win them back? I need to do something that wins them back with my winning philosophy."

God. This is exactly as bad as I thought it would be. No, it's worse. He's worse than I thought he was when I was high. He smells worse than a bus station urinal. He smells like the inside of a port-o-potty at some drunk festival where it's really hot outside and it's the end of a day where everybody's been puking their beer guts out all day long with diarrhea from spoiled hot dogs.

5:01 AM: I'm bleary. My head bobs. I keep dozing off. What a relief if I could snuff him out and go to sleep. If he was a normal cellmate I would have slept all night.

Sleep? I miss my bed; my clean, soft sheets, my extra pillow, my own room. It's dark and quiet and nobody comes in. Just the thought of it all and I can…No! I catch myself. Keep these eyes open. The maniac will flip out if I'm not paying attention.

"It was part of the rush of pleasure — pleasure seeking behavior. It's just like a person having a drink. It's pleasurable getting what you want. I had one girlfriend who said I worked too hard at having fun; she said this as we were mainlining cocaine. That's dangerous, Danny, because you can get diseases. After a while, I ended up using up all my veins and that happened just as crack came around. So, first I was snorting it, and then I was shooting it, and then I was smoking it."

I will never speak to Captain again. Even if it's a Friday night and I'm facing a whole weekend without pot and I know he's on The Ave on his perch, I refuse to go to him.

Maybe I'll send a friend.

5:22 AM: "We holed up in a motel room playing cards and shooting coke. By the end of the weekend, I had broken through to the other side. I saw lights in the forest which was clearly a UFO. I wanted to walk into the woods and meet up with the aliens because I knew they were here to make contact with humans, and I'm a friendly guy, so I knew I should be the one to welcome them."

My eyesight is completely blurry. The pencils are now nubs and won't write anything anymore. My kites are filled with spider-looking chicken scratch. There's one kite I can actually make out. I wrote it at 3:03 AM. It was a magical time, so Captain insisted I make this list.

1. KNOW YOUR CUSTOMER
2. ACT LIKE YOU'RE MARRIED
3. KNOW WHEN YOU'RE DIVORCED
4. BUY BOOZE EVEN IF YOU DON'T DRINK (for the ladies)
5. WATCH FOR SIGNS FROM SPIRITS
6. LEARN HOW TO READ CARDS
7. FIND A PLACE TO SLEEP
8. YOU CAN GET WARM IF YOU'RE DRY, BUT YOU CAN'T GET DRY IF YOU'RE WET
9. CHOOSE YOUR FRIENDS CAREFULLY
10. RECOGNIZE AN UNDERCOVER COP

5:55 AM: Three of the same number. What did he say about that? Beware? Does that mean beware of what he's saying, or beware of him, or of someone else coming in? The guard? Beware of leaving? How do you figure out what you're supposed to beware of?

"The angels told me I am entitled to compensation from the government. It appears that our arrangement here tonight is going to be my payment. All things being equal, it seems like it's not an unfair exchange. Wouldn't you say, Danny?"

"Oh…" I haven't spoken out loud for about ninety minutes. My tongue feels like it's covered with a stiff sock from a dirty pile of laundry. "Definitely seems fair."

"Why? Why does it seem fair to you?"

"Well…" It's like the time I fell asleep in class. Captain's raising his brows at me as though he expects me to immediately chime in. Like this has been some kind of an equal conversation all night long and my eyes aren't glued to the back of my head. He expects an answer.

I make a neat pile out of the kites so he thinks I'm being very thoughtful. "The angels wouldn't tell you if it was not fair." He absorbs my statement. I'm speaking his language. I guess I sound like I've been alert.

"But why did the spirits let it happen in the first place? It was done without my consent. Without my consent!" His voice is shrill. "I was a kid, Danny! I was just an innocent child!"

I've been almost dozing off for hours, but I don't think I fell totally asleep. I don't remember him saying anything about his childhood. He digs his claws into his temples. He scrunches up his whole face.

He's dark again, darker than ever. Shit. Shit.

Captain bellows, "THE FREEDOM OF INFORMATION ACT!"

I jet straight up. The kites scatter. Now I'm awake. Fully. On high alert.

Captain throws wild punches at no one, "IT'S NOT TOP SECRET ANYMORE!"

Cover my head — race to my corner — hide the pencil nubs in my palm — in case I need something sharp to stab his face.

I twist to Beef. He doesn't even lift his head from his files. Unbelievable!

"I know! I know what was done to me!" Captain rages in every direction. "I know what you assholes did to those of us who could not fight back!" Captain's maniacal eyes shift to me.

My heart pounds in my ears. Oh, no. He can't turn his fury on me. Please! I imitate my mother's soothing voice, "Captain, its okay."

"Those are the words the CIA used in their documentation. *People who could not fight back!* Prostitutes, mental patients, prisoners, drug addicts, other CIA employees, and children, Danny!" He's mad at the CIA, and not at me. Not at me. Oh, thank God. "CHILDREN! LIKE ME!"

Gotta get him down. Carefully. I'm so close to getting out of here. This can't turn into Reality Rush Number Three. "Kite's in the slot, Captain. I signed it. It's just sitting there, waiting for the guards to take it whenever they get to it. Could be hours from now. They're just doing their time, in their government job. My signature has to be worth something. You said so yourself. They'll recognize that."

"Recognize. Yes." He looks at my feet, my shoulders, and my face; like he's seeing me again for the first time. "My God. It's astounding." His eyes well up.

Wait. Wait. Is he going to cry?

Captain's shoulders slump. His arms go limp. His pain spills out in wet sobs, rinsing his anger down the sunken ravines that are his cheeks. His drowning eyes reach out to me like he's fallen into a swamp and cannot swim. He wants me to save him.

I didn't expect this. He's like a scared little kid. Strangely, I want to help him from whatever he's tangled up in. I feel like I should pull him out and make him feel better, like my dad did when I'd have a nightmare.

I relax my grip on my nub. "What did you find out from the Freedom of Information Act?" I stand straight. Come out of my corner. I'm the adult who is unafraid and in control. "You want to tell me about that, Captain? Tell me. I'm listening."

He wipes his eyes with his rough sleeves. "Our government is so cruel, Danny."

"What did they do?"

"You ever hear of Project Artichoke? Or Project Bluebird?"

6:08 AM: "No, Captain. Tell me." I sit on the floor so he'll sit on the bench. He drops on his haunches and hangs his head. His tears drip like rain drops slipping off the edge of a freeway.

"I looked this up in the library. For about twenty years, our government allowed the CIA to conduct secret experiments to brainwash people. They gave all kinds of drugs to people who had NO IDEA what was happening to them and then they tried to erase their memories afterward. God." His snot glistens under his nose like a trail left by a wet slug.

I grab the roll of toilet paper off the floor. "Here, Captain."

"They addicted people to morphine and heroin to see if they were more pliable when they were in withdrawal. They gave them LSD. People had hallucinations. They killed themselves! Jumped out windows! One guy who headed the program hated what he was doing and wanted to tell the world. Just days after he quit, he was murdered by the CIA! They murdered him to protect their dirty secrets!"

"I've never heard of this."

"Welcome to the illicit underworld of our government! We live in a non-spiritual world, and I guess people have to do things like this to live in it. We live in a world filled with consumers. The guy's family — the one the CIA murdered — sued and got money from the government. Now I deserve mine too."

"So…you think you were experimented on?"

"Think? I know I was, Danny! I was in the hospital not thirty miles from a military base in Aberdeen, Maryland." He mops his face and blows his nose.

I'm not telling him, but my family lived in Aberdeen when my dad worked as a doctor for the military.

"The CIA did their experiments in a bunch of locations, including hospitals. I have no recollection of my time in the hospital, and I remember everything, Danny. I know I've done a lot of drugs, but I don't forget anything! They put a chip in me and they erased my memory! They've been following me for all these years! They spotted me as a special person when I was a kid, and they tried to control me, to get into my head. Now that I'm older, I'm more valuable to them because I can communicate with the spirits. But I demand to be compensated for my suffering. My years of suffering."

He unrolls more toilet paper. He looks so defeated. I'm not inspired to even think anything sarcastic about his conspiracy theories. He's making me too sad.

"How come you went to the hospital?"

Shreds of toilet paper stick to his face. "Dehydration, I think."

"How old were you?"

"Seven. Eight."

I just remembered. I was also put in the hospital at that age.

When we lived in Aberdeen.

6:12 AM: It's freaky how we were both in the hospital at the same age in the same city. That is just a weird coincidence. I've met born-again Christians who say there's no such thing as coincidences. Mormons must also believe in some kind of help from God. Why go to church if God doesn't want to communicate with us or help us?

I heard someone say that coincidences are God's way of staying anonymous. So…if He put us together, what is His plan?

Maybe the reason I got busted was because God wants me to help Captain somehow. Like our being alone in this jail cell will be some kind of spiritual tuning for him in the same way Captain described tuning a radio. Maybe I can help to synchronize him with a better wave length of thinking.

Captain blows his nose. "So that's the reason I'm homeless and addicted to drugs."

"You think it's all because of Project Blue Bird?"

"Yes. I was persecuted. I am persecuted. I'm being held back by the government." Captain wraps his finger in a piece of toilet paper and wedges out his gooey leftover boogers with it. Weird that someone so dirty would be careful that way. That's the way my mom used to wipe her nose too. "They ruined my life by messing me up when I was a kid and they've been keeping me down all these years, but not anymore, Danny. Not after tonight. You know how it's always the poor people who become professional boxers? They beat the shit out of each other for the entertainment of the rich. That's all I am to them. That's all both of us are tonight, Danny. We're just fodder for the government. Entertainment for the rich."

"But our government wouldn't…"

"I just told you what they did to me, and thousands of others! We can't get our lives back. It's their fault! I'm lucky I'm even alive!" He throws his wadded-up tissues into a pile in the corner. "Have you ever heard of the Illuminati?"

"Yeah, I think so. But..."

"They control things like who gets to become lawyers. They decide who gets to become Secretary of State. There are Masonic temples in every major city." He picks at the tissue fuzzies stuck on his face. "These are real buildings, Danny. I'm sure you've seen them. A bunch of hypocrites! They espouse traditional values but go have affairs on their wives. The Masons have double standards just like our whole country! The rich can get away with taking drugs if they want to. But if you're a poor person doing drugs, you have police officers going after you and throwing you in jail. I didn't do anything wrong by doing drugs, because lots of rich people were doing them and were getting away with it! So, if a kid has parents who are Masons, he has a chance of getting a good job but a poor person wouldn't have that same advantage. It's a double standard! It's not fair! You ever look closely at a dollar bill?"

"Not really. But what does all that..."

"Look at it! There are Masonic symbols all over it! You know the eye on top of the unfinished pyramid?"

"I don't know, maybe?"

"Give me a pencil." He motions for me to hurry up. I hand him a nub. Maybe I shouldn't have given it to him. He's getting worked up again. He motions to the kites that are still all over the floor. "Those are all filled up?"

"Yeah."

Captain unrolls some toilet paper on the bench and draws on it. It's a faint drawing and the paper is torn, but I can sort of make it out. He exclaims, "It's the All-Seeing Eye! It's encased in a triangle, which represents the unfinished pyramid and reminds us of the immortality of the soul. It's a reminder that we will complete the capstones of our earthly labors in heaven. See?" He flaps his knuckles at his drawing of the eye in the triangle. "This is from our United States Treasury! If the Masons can influence what's printed on a U.S. dollar bill, the

Masons can influence who is a member of the CIA and who the CIA is watching!"

He punctuates this by slamming the nub on the bench. It jars me into attention. God. What the hell is real in what he's saying? What is just crazy talk? I've seen Masonic Temples. They're everywhere, and I heard somewhere some of our Founding Fathers were Masons. But seriously? Do they really control every single stupid job and who gets picked for it? Everyone knows there's a CIA, but did they really do drug experiments on people? That's hard to believe. But, even if they did, was Captain actually one of them? Really? It's pathetic he's so certain of it. If Captain's been to jail eighteen times he must have seen a psychiatrist sometime in there. Why didn't any of them help him?

Then again, I'm not sure I buy the whole "getting therapy" business. Some doctors are just full of shit and want to take your money. Like the shrink my parents forced me to go to when I was in grade school.

We were living in a tough neighborhood in Seattle and I hung out with a pack of thieves who had schemes to steal magazines, toys and candy. They even teamed up to rip off the local Laundromat. One kid would keep an eye out while another kid crawled across the floor and snuck into the safe to steal rolls of dimes, nickels, and quarters. They never got busted.

I began stealing in the third or fourth grade and actually got to be pretty good at it. It was a lot of fun until the fifth grade when I got caught at the neighborhood drug store. It was kinda funny because I went in thinking I was being clever by wearing my scout uniform which made me look trustworthy. While the pharmacist was busy with another customer, I casually wriggled three pieces of licorice into my front pocket. As I headed for the door, the pharmacist's wife grabbed me with her blood red fingernails. Because of that wiry-haired ugly bitch, all my good times ended and my parents sent me to see a psychiatrist.

All the shrink and I ever did was play games. That's it. I don't know why we played them or what we even talked about. I do remember I didn't want anyone from school to know I saw a psychiatrist. But here was my mom coming at least once a week to pull me out of class. And the kids began to wonder where I was going.

They could be pretty mean, and I didn't want to get a nickname or anything. But there's nothing worse than people thinking you're crazy, so every week I had to come up with some new story to tell my friends about where she was taking me. One lie I made up was I had to go to the doctor because I swallowed a large piece of gum and it got stuck in my throat. This one kid laughed and said I was really going to a psychiatrist. I froze up because I thought he had found me out. It turned out he was only joking but it still made me sick inside.

There was a magazine stand located near the psychiatrist's office. My mom would drop me off there so I could buy a pack of gum before I went in for my appointment. Later on, I'd triple my money by selling the extra pieces to my friends at school. Eventually, I started stealing the packs of gum and it became my own personal game. When we moved to our new house about a year later, my parents finally stopped taking me to the appointments. This was a huge relief because I didn't want to have to come up with stories to tell my new friends. Thankfully, no one ever found out at either school. Going to a psychiatrist was, and is, my one darkly held secret.

That shrink must have cost my parents a lot of money but I can't think of one good thing that came from me going to see him. I guess even if someone had tried to get mental help for Captain, it might have been as much of a waste of time for him as it was for me. Still, I was just a kid getting a thrill from doing something naughty. But Captain's really suffering, and it's hard to watch him.

Maybe God wants me to help him by telling him he can still make something out of his life. He should put the same energy that he has on his Urban Bullshit-Whatever-Engineer and go sell some cars or something.

He hands me the eye in the triangle. "Here. Keep it."

I take it along with the nub. "Even with the Masons and Illuminati, do you wish you had tried a regular job? Seems like you're good at business."

"Danny, people are jealous."

"Of who?"

He smiles broadly. His smattering of teeth jut out like cigarette butts stuffed randomly in an ashtray. "Me!"

"They are?"

"Are you kidding? Yes!" Captain gets on the floor and picks up the kites. "All those working stiffs see me out and about having a good time. They question their own choice of signing on for the nine-to-five life with a wife and kids. It's real easy to do sales on a Monday night, because the stiffs have just gotten back to work and really need something to look forward to. So my role has been a virtuous one. Of course, the problem was always that they see me." He stands up on his knees and holds his arms out like *ta-da*. "I've chosen the path they were too afraid to take: the yellow brick road of the good life, the party life. And they are jealous."

All the kites collected, Captain hands me his pile. He seems more relaxed, less paranoid. Maybe he's coming down from his high. Maybe he'll accept some advice from me and I can do something good before 8:00 AM. Then again, after all those years of drug abuse, can he ever truly sober up? His face looks like slabs of beef jerky that have been peppered and smoked in illegal substances for thirty years. I say, "Thanks."

"But, to answer your question, before I started dealing drugs I did try to get a normal job. But no one would hire me." Captain uses the bench to push himself up. "So I got a case of *The Fuck-its.*"

6:20 AM: Six and two. Captain would say if you multiply them, they would equal twelve.

Captain holds his lower back like an old man. "Can't stop looking at the clock, can you, Danny? That could be construed as obsessive-compulsive behavior. But tell me, since you're wrapped up in it, what do you gather from 6:20?"

"Uh…that you would tell me about the Twelve Apostles."

"Excellent. But I will meet you and raise you one better: the number eight."

"Why? What's significant about the number eight?"

"Danny! Put an eight on its side. Oh yeah. It's the symbol for infinity." His eyes dance. "Infinity. Which is fascinating because you're being released at 8:00 AM." He whispers, "What ever could be the message behind that numerological coincidence?"

Maybe infinite possibilities? The infinity of time? What does he mean? No! Forget it! I'm not going let him trap me in his sticky spider web thinking!

He tilts toward me and points to the ceiling where the CIA supposedly has their hidden camera. "What do they have planned for you at 8:00 AM? Could it be…"

"No clue! But I do want to know what The Fuck-its are."

"Oh." His eyes bow out. He bends over to pick up his pile of used tissues. "Well, look, I don't come from a family of Masons or Illuminati. I couldn't compete with the rich kids and their trust funds. And then my fiancé…"

He holds the tissues in his arms. He can't seem to finish that thought. Don't want him to go on anymore about the ladies or Social Lubricants so I change the subject. "Do you have family? Couldn't they…?"

Captain shrugs, "My mom put down first and last deposit on three apartments but I lost all those places — and she also bought me three cars — but I sold them for drugs. After that, she refused to help me anymore. She said she'd had enough of me. Her only son."

"Is there anyone else?"

"I stay with my sister. Sometimes." He throws the tissues in the toilet one by one. "So I had to find my own place. Outside. It was harder than you think. All the overpasses were taken already because every homeless person wants shelter in a city where it rains almost every damned day. But when it's windy, forget it. There's no way to stay dry. When the rain pelts sideways, the plywood walls around my bed don't help much." He motions a tissue at me, "Even still. It's a good camp. When I was looking for a place, I ran across a dude who had dug himself a trench, like a foxhole. He sat there in his hole, smoking rolled up cigarettes. He had hundreds of butts stuck in the hill all around him. It was just saddening to me that he'd made his life like that. I made a solemn promise to take care of my own place. I put a tarp underneath the cushions I slept on and used it to cover the hill where the dirt came down so my clothes and hair wouldn't get dirty. I couldn't shower that much, but I wore a knit cap and I never pissed in my pants or anything, and I didn't get that close to people where they could smell me, anyway. Even though my clothes were sticky, crusty and stale, they were drab in color, like what everyone else in Seattle wears. They didn't have holes in them — like some of those homeless teenagers I came across — so I think I did a pretty good job of not looking like a homeless person." He throws in the last tissue. "I worked in the center of the city and everybody needed to know I was the man who knew what was going on. Ergo, I took great pains to not appear homeless. People weren't going to talk to me or buy from me if I had a sleeping bag strapped on my back."

How can he not know how bad he looks and stinks? Before he can do anything positive with his life, he'd have to be shaved, fumigated, and sandblasted with Borax.

Captain opens his empty hands. "Imagine if Mary, Mother of Jesus, gave up on her only son." He stares at the glob of tissues in the bowl and says, "My parents gave up on me right after the thing with my fiancé, and I decided I might as well go live outside and do drugs. That, Danny, is what you call The Fuck-its'." He stomps the handle, flushing the toilet paper away.

I wait until it's quiet. He's still there like he's waiting for the tissues to come back. "What kind of a job did you apply for?"

"Legal work."

I raise my eyebrows. I imagine him, completely out of his mind, walking into a law firm, meeting the fancy secretary at the front desk, and handing her his resume written on a kite he swiped from jail. Security must have thrown him out on his ass. I ask innocently, "You wanted to be a legal assistant?"

"I would have taken any kind of work that was related to the law...just until I could practice law myself."

"Got it." I cover my smirk, in case he turns around. I don't want to be mean.

He lifts his head. "Actually, I did get a job with one sleazy attorney." Captain walks over to the guard's window. "He used to drive around town with a junky in his passenger seat, trying to find somebody who was driving an expensive car. One fat cat he preyed on looked just like our guard here." He nods his chin to Beefsteak who's dumping powdered cream into his Styrofoam cup. "Coffee. I'd like some. Why cream and no sugar? Is he giving a signal to the CIA?"

"I've never had coffee."

"I didn't start drinking it until I had to take an early morning bankruptcy class." Captain leans against the window and faces me. "Anyway, when the sleazeball would spot a nice car, he'd cut over to their lane and accelerate right in front of the guy, and then he'd slam it into reverse, right into the fat cat's car. He'd make it look like a rear-end accident. Then he'd have the junky he was driving around with file a medical complaint against the rich guy's insurance company. I kept the corporate books for this crook and had to back date documents for him. I couldn't believe I had gone to law school for that kind of thievery. He was a joke of a lawyer. Eventually, he fired me because I had a terrible attitude about his work. But getting laid off gave me more time to study for the bar."

Back up a second. I sit up straight. "Uh, what did you — did you say you studied for the bar?"

He stretches his arms above his head. "Yes."

"So you went to law school?"

"That's when I started drinking coffee. In bankruptcy class."

Maybe in his delusional brain he mistook what was actually a prisoner rehabilitation class to be what he thought was law school. "Where did you go to law school?"

"I graduated from USC."

"The University of…"

"Southern California. Yes."

"Law school?"

He yawns, "Yes."

No fucking way. This is just more of his kooky horseshit about hidden cameras, a trip to Mars and Government Artichoke.

How can I help him if he's lying? Come on. Here I am trying to be a good Christian and, for once in my life, trying to help a fellow human being because I feel bad for him, and he was crying, and whatever. Maybe something bad did happen to him in his childhood. Probably a lot bad has happened to him in his life.

But he's purposely lying by showing a fake portrait of himself! That is bullshit. I want to see his paint and his brushes. I don't care if he's loony. I clear my throat, "Seems to me you'd still have a pretty good chance of finding a job in some kind of company, even with the government being after you. That is, if you actually had a law degree from USC."

"But I didn't pass the bar."

"Because of the Illuminati?"

"And the Masons."

"Right."

"There were some other things."

"You mean, like The Others who are watching us?"

"Yes."

So he wants me to think his portrait is one of success until the Masons and Illuminati came and slashed it to pieces. When he lies like this, he must think he can make me respect him, or he's trying to impress me. Whatever he's trying to do, it's obvious he'd rather point the paint brush at anyone else for his failure, instead of the painter himself.

Becoming a lawyer takes hard work and focus. You have to put in the time and sacrifice. Like me. I'm studying hard, hitting the books. My goal to be a lawyer is set in stone. No wavering. No cheating. Good grades are earned. My parents would never allow me to blame the boogie man because I blew my chances. Just like they're making me face up to my consequences by forcing me spend the night in jail — which is way, way, way, way, way too harsh.

When Captain casually lies about something that is already taking a lot of sacrifice from my life, it really pisses me off. I can't become a lawyer without taking the bar exam. The only thing Captain is willing to make any kind of sacrifice for is getting high.

6:32 AM: I watch the third hand click the seconds by. Countdown is now one hour, twenty-eight minutes. I tried to help him. But now I'm done. I can't wait until he's out of my life.

Captain muses, "It's 6:32. Good number. Three and two are two prime numbers. The Masons use thirty-two, which is a reversal of twenty-three: a favorite of the Illuminati. And of course, there's *twenty-three skidoo!*"

I yawn really loudly, "Really?"

"It means: 'You're bad luck. It's time to get out'. Twenty-three is from *A Tale of Two Cities*. At the end of the book, they were bringing people up by the hundreds to chop off their heads. So this character was number twenty-three when he gets the guillotine." Captain uses his long-nailed finger to slice across his neck. "*Skidoo* is like skedaddle."

"Hm."

Captain gets up. "In honor of the numerical significance to the Masons and Illuminati, I will tell you about the other things I meant, other than The Others. The things that went down right after law school: my girlfriend, my parents, the bar exam prep course."

"Uh-huh." Christ, maybe I can sleep with my eyes open.

He slides his back down the wall and stretches his legs out before him. Here we go, settling in to listen to a Dickens novel. At least I don't have to take notes.

6:34 AM: Captain leans his head next to some gang scrawl. He sighs and begins. "Danny, I graduated from law school in the bottom third of my class and I could not figure out why I did so poorly. Of course, I since found out it was because of the chip the CIA put in me but, at the time, I felt terrible. Anyway, all my friends were taking a prep course to study for the bar exam, but I went on a vacation to Europe with my girlfriend.

She and I were living together in LA. She expected me to propose on the trip, but I didn't because I didn't have a job yet. After we got back, my daily life was completely different. I was used to being with friends and going to classes, but I wasn't taking the prep course, and my girlfriend went to work, so I was all alone in our apartment every day. I couldn't stand it and went to the beach to study until the time came to take the bar. While I was waiting to get the results, I took a minimum wage job because I couldn't find a law job for anything, because of the Masons and the Illuminati. One day, I came home from work and found my girlfriend had moved out. There was no way I could afford the apartment on my own, I was out of money, and my parents weren't giving me any more. I called my mom and asked her if I could move home. I flew back to Washington and got drunk with a lady in the back of the plane." Captain snorts at the memory and flashes me his ashtray smile. "Social Lubricant, Danny. The laaaadies love it."

Through a fake smile I say, "Got it."

He shifts his boney butt on the hard floor and continues. "Since I moved to another state, I had to start all over and take the bar exam there. See, Danny, the chip was holding me down by making me go back to Washington. Let me tell you, life in Seattle turned out to be utter shit. I took a job at a telemarketing company which made things even shittier. It was a real fall from grace, from being the golden boy at USC to a telemarketer whose job description didn't even require a high school education. I called to find out about my results on the California bar and they said I passed the first part. It made me feel great, so I studied really hard for the Washington bar, but I ended up failing it miserably. Wanting to try again, I finally got to take a review course. By then, I was hanging out with an old friend who became a cocaine dealer. So while I was studying to take the Washington bar for the second time, I was also doing lines."

He's silent. Tense, he tightly weaves his fingers together. "I didn't pass it the second time, Danny. I missed it. Again. By four. Fucking. Points." He flashes four fingers at me. "Four points, Danny! Passing score was 1240. I was at 1236. It was my second F! I never, ever got an F before this. I maybe had one D in my entire academic life. But I never took the bar again. If only I knew then what I know now: it was what they had planned for me all along."

God. Oh my God. He really did get his law degree.

I never knew you could flunk out after you graduated from law school. I heard passing the bar was hard, but I just didn't think much about what happens if you don't pass it. I feel stupid thinking about this possibility right now for the very first time. He went to school for seven years after high school. After all that money spent on tuition, all those hours of studying, he has nothing. He'll never be a lawyer. What a waste.

I don't know what to say to him. "Shit." That's all I can come up with.

"Yep." He gets up. "Shit. Good word. It came from the times when they used to transport manure for fertilizer. If the crates were stowed away in the bottom of a hold the gases built up and created a hazard with the lanterns. Hence: 'Ship High In Transport' and 'S.H.I.T' was stamped on the crates."

"Is that where you went to undergrad? At USC?"

"No. I went to the University of Washington. Right next to The Ave. My perch. I know the campus inside out. I slept there sometimes."

"Where?"

"U-dub" campus. The best place is the Mechanical Engineering Building. It is open the latest and the longest: 6:00 AM to 11:00 PM. They have nice, comfortable chairs. I'd go in there in the morning, push four chairs together and fall asleep." Captain rubs his neck. "Could use those big chairs right now."

My whole body agrees. "Yeah. Sucks."

"After I slept for a few hours, a security guard would wake me up and get me moving on. They tried to have me banned from campus once, but the judge wouldn't allow it. They have one area on the grass where there are three heat vents. Hot air blows up and it gets warm, but if it looked like I was curling up to sleep over a manhole, they would tell me to move along."

He sleeps outside on the same campus where he got his degree? How can he stand to be there? I ask, "What about your camp?"

"Sometimes I didn't feel like crossing the freeway. Remember I told you about the pillar that kept me from falling to my death onto the I-5? Well, there's a three foot wide path around that pillar. I had to edge along it to get into my camp. When I say there was nothing, I mean no-thing, between me and that sixty foot drop. I never looked down when I squeezed by. That's probably the reason nobody else claimed it before me. Because nobody else had the guts to get in and out of there. Well, okay, I did bring four or five women there. Maybe six. I always helped them safely across the freeway."

It's hard for me to believe that he'd get nothing — absolutely nothing — from all that education. I shake my head and scoff, "You're telling me the only job in the world you could get was dealing drugs? That was your only choice?"

"No, I got jobs at a t-shirt business and a video dating service. But they didn't pay very much. My rent was eating up most of my earnings. Plus, I took out a student loan in law school. I had that bill coming in every month. It was $480 every month. I couldn't pay it on minimum wage, so I defaulted on it. A lot of bad shit happens when you default on a student loan, Danny. Your credit is ruined. Messes up a lot of stuff. And then my fiancé got pregnant."

"Thought you said you didn't want to get married until you had a job."

"That was my girlfriend in LA. The one I got engaged to was later on, after I came back to Seattle. That was a coincidence. I was leaving Denny's at 2:00 AM and ran into my old girlfriend from high school. She was on her way to the police station to get her friend out of jail. It wasn't long before I proposed. She was an accounts receiver and had good credit so she bought her own engagement ring. Then she got pregnant but we decided she should have an abortion. I just wasn't ready to live that responsible life. I still wanted the footloose and fancy-free lifestyle. All that happened about the same time I lost my last apartment. And that's when it happened."

"What?"

"The Fuck-its. Ya know? FUCK! IT! Who gives a shit?"

He's pretty casual about something so serious. I wonder if his fiancé gave a shit about the baby or about Captain. He must have looked different back then. Still, it's hard to imagine what woman would ever want to marry him.

He stands up and goes to the guard's window. "One time, I stood outside a Masonic Temple on Greenlake. I was holding a map of Las Vegas in my hands. I figured the capitol for the Illuminati must be in Sin City. I wanted to break a window of the temple." He puts his nose and an open palm on the window and eyeballs everything in Beefy's station. "Wanted to get inside to find an answer. Desperate for any answer about life and how mine turned out like this. I didn't go through with it because I was afraid I'd get arrested and then I wouldn't get my crack."

"Crack."

"Yeah. Like I said, it was always cocaine." In a monotone, Captain says, "One hit and it was okay I was Chosen. Didn't need to have a different life. Didn't matter if my family didn't talk to me or I didn't have a wife and kids. Didn't have to be an NBA star or Rep of the Month or an associate in a law firm. I didn't have to do anything but get high and I felt incredible. It was that easy."

"It doesn't sound like it to me, Captain. A real job would have been a lot easier. Did you ever look into social work? Or teaching?"

"Danny, I get messages from the Holy Spirit." He rolls his eyes. "Or did you forget that already? It's in that pile of notes, kid."

"I didn't forget, but how could you think God would want you to sleep under a freeway?"

"Yeah, there were times when, at the end of a day, when I passed by those big houses lit up with families inside. I wondered why I didn't deserve that too. But then the angels told me I was living the right way. So I made the most of my camp. It was mine. Private. No one stepping over me. Bare-assed naked, cozy and comfortable in my thick sleeping bag."

"God wouldn't…"

He cuts me off, "God wouldn't *what*? Look what happened to Jesus! Job! Joseph Smith was murdered! There's no wavering when God chooses you! Because, Jesus, Danny, if you're Chosen, you do what the angels tell you to do. What the hell would have happened to Christianity if John the Baptist ignored his calling because he wanted to buy a house and start a family? Or if Joseph Smith became a social worker or a teacher? We would not have Christianity or the Mormon Church today! Have you ever heard the Mormon story?"

"Yeah."

"Then you know that an angel appeared before Joseph Smith right here in our country in 1823. Not thousands of years ago in Jerusalem. Don't you get it? I'm exactly like Joseph Smith. And I'm Mormon too."

I would never have guessed he was a Mormon. Except that, earlier, he said something about words of wisdom. Still, it's not that big of a deal. There are a lot of Mormons in Seattle. Why not a crazy Mormon? He probably converted, but wound up scaring the shit out of everyone and they had to excommunicate him. But no way am I telling him I grew up LDS. I don't need him going off on that one.

"Are you familiar with Joseph Smith, Danny?"

I say only, "Yes." Before he can prod me for more, I ask, "Were you converted by a missionary or something?"

Captain beams, "I've been Mormon all my life. I was raised in it. I grew up going to church four times a week. They taught us that we were all special people. Chosen people. And when we die, we'll be gods of our own planets. Joseph Smith was visited by an angel named Moroni…"

"Right. I know."

Captain whips his hands in front of his face. "Well, an angel appeared before *me* and told *me* what to do! Maybe a Catholic or a Jew would be freaked out if that happened to them, but it made perfect sense to me because of Joseph Smith. It still does. I want to be sure it makes sense to you too."

I ask, "Are your parents Mormon?"

"They were both raised in the church. They met at BYU and had a Temple marriage." Typical scenario. "They stopped taking us to church when I was about twelve and never said why. We went from being in a church where we stored a year's worth of canned food so we'd be ready when Jesus returned to earth, because the stores won't be open. Where people fasted once a month so they could stand up in front of everybody and give their personal testimony. We'd have Mormon missionaries over for dinner. We'd pray before meals. My dad would pray in the car before we'd take a road trip. Then we went to nothing. Nothing! No church. Without any explanation! But I had bought into everything the church taught me. I believed all of it! And then, one day, the church and everything we did around it was gone. Just gone. I was so confused. Sad. We weren't doing all the activities we used to do with the church like scouts and summer camp. It was so fun. But no one explained anything to me."

It was the same way for me.

Captain rears his head toward me. He's got that ominous look. No. Not again.

From under his deep brow, his steely eyes drill a hole into me. His voice lowers an octave. "That's why I'm explaining everything to you, Danny. So you have direction when you get out of here at the infinite time of 8:00 AM. That is, until you get arrested again."

6:59 AM: Lighten him up! Only one hour and one minute to go! I give a funny wave of my hands with an exaggerated laugh, "Ha! No, no, no, Captain! I am never going to jail again!"

He breaks a smile, "Oh yeah? Good luck with that, Rocket Man. Either you're quitting pot or it's being legalized or you'll magically dodge the all-seeing eye of the law. But now that you've signed and deposited that kite, I don't see any of these things happening."

I cheerily point out: "I'll fight to make it legal!"

"Right on! That's what I was going to do!" He puts out his hand for another hi-five. I do it. Good, good. I moved him past doomsday. He makes a point back: "But, ya know you'll never be able to work for the government now that you've got a misdemeanor."

"Is that true?"

"No FBI, no CIA, no county prosecutor's office. You'll never get a government job where you do twenty years and get pension and benefits. The CIA came to USC to interview; it actually looked pretty cool but it was not an option."

"But I thought you said you were hiding from the CIA."

"Did you lose where we are in the story? I was not aware at that point I was Chosen! It's been a hard fucking life since I realized they were following me. Subsisting on locusts! That's the problem with being John the Baptist, Danny. Nothing ever changes."

I shake my head and say, "Not true. You can change."

He rolls his shoulders back and holds his head high. "Yes. Yes, I can. You are one astute observer, Danny. Because you are absolutely correct. It is time for me to live the straight life. Give up all this drug business. I was not ready until tonight. Until I met you."

His puts his hand out for me to shake. Ruddy, weathered, dirty, with thick soot under the nails: a hand so obviously in need of help.

And he says I'm helping him. Wow.

I don't fake laugh or smile. I'm moved inside. Truly moved.

I look up into his eyes and see another human soul.

There. Put it there. I stand up and take his hand. Shake. His knuckles wrap tight around my hand, crushing it. His palm is scratchy and calloused. But my heart is soft.

Oh, man! I feel good! Now it makes sense to me why people go around helping others. Preaching and getting people to convert. I am doing God's will by changing this man's life.

I cover our gripped hands with my other hand. My accomplishment washes over me like a baptism. I say, "Glad to hear it, Captain. There's so much you can do."

7:01 AM: We release our hands and stand there a second. It's awkward. There's nowhere to look.

"Yeah. Big changes!" He cracks his knuckles. "It's good timing because, like I said, if I get convicted once more, it's three strikes and I'm out. Once more and I'll go to prison. Not just juvenile-boot-camp-jail: I'll go to hard-time prison."

"Just so I know, Captain, what did I say that made you change your mind?"

"Nothing. You signed the kite. That's all. The kite that said you're taking over for me so I get to go free. That's my payment for sharing my words of wisdom with you." He bows his head to me. "Thank you, Danny. I'm grateful for the compensation."

"Uh..." I guffaw, "What am I taking over?"

"I told you to read the contract very carefully before you signed it. My post on The Ave, my customers, my work with the spirits. The CIA will be watching you instead of me. Sorry, though, you're wrong about not getting arrested again. The cops will be all over you."

"I couldn't read it..." There's that feeling again of the tiny claws scurrying across the back of my neck. It makes me shiver.

"Hey, ya know what I call it? When the cops snap those handcuffs on your wrists?"

I shake my head.

"*Reality Bracelets.*"

What? What did he just say? I brush my neck. I know it's impossible, but I can't help but feel like rodents are crawling all over my neck and back.

"Yeah. It's like you're getting high, laughing with some ladies and then — BAM! You get those Reality Bracelets cracked on your wrists and you gotta come down fast, straighten up and deal with reality."

My insides scream. It's like I've slipped underneath a manhole. It's dark and no one can hear me. He continues: "A lot of things were like that in my life. Like when I found out I was Chosen. I used to have life goals. A list of goals I had written down on a piece of paper I carried with me everywhere I went. But God laughed at my list. The Holy Spirit showed me I was Chosen and I couldn't get out of it. That was a Reality Rush of epic proportions."

Trapped under my manhole, his words come at me like flying squirrels landing on my head. Their pin-like paws and furry tails crawl in my hair, scratch my face, and ferret down the insides of my jumpsuit. I hear myself say, "What?"

"Oh, what's a Reality Rush? I made that one up when I was about your age. It's when life stops you dead." His face scrunches and his eyes well up. He pinches the bridge of his nose. "Like when my fiancé got an abortion. My biggest regret: telling her to get an abortion."

I swallow. "What — uh, what was your fiancé's name?"

He sighs. He wipes his tears with his fingers and then on his jumpsuit. His voice rounds like an echo, not from him, but from the sewer of my own soul. His lips form, "Lynette."

Blood surges all around, drowning me in the manhole. It's dark, soft, and floaty. A blanket of warm fur caresses under my skin and oozes through my veins. Everything goes black.

When we moved to Bellevue in sixth grade, I made a new group of friends from the neighborhood. We'd walk to school together, eat lunch together. One of them was a kid named Starky. He came from a Catholic family of six kids. He went to scouts with me and we got to go on camp-outs and hikes. We learned how to set up tents and build a campfire. We earned merit badges for archery, leather working, canoeing. Starky was the first kid who ever asked me if I smoked pot.

But over the years, as I've gotten to know Starky better, I can tell there's something off about him. I can't put my finger on it. He says weird shit about masturbating, things like that. If he wasn't an old friend from the neighborhood I would stop talking to him. Steve and I put up with him mainly because he's a good skier.

Starky and I are in the same biology class at school. We're studying the physiology of the brain. Last week, Starky told me he thought the TV was talking to him directly. To him and to no one else. I couldn't believe he would admit that to anyone.

And to me? We're just casual friends. Like I said, I'll never, ever, tell him, or anyone else, that my parents made me go to a psychiatrist, even though it was several years ago.

WHAM! The back of my head bonks like I've been hit with a drain pipe. The soft, furry blanket that caressed my veins rips off me like a security guard shaking me awake from my comfortable place. Out of my bloody sewer, I gasp for air.

I'm on the floor. Captain's face blurs into focus. He's over me. His hair droops over my face like cobwebs.

"Danny? You hit your head!"

Ow. Oh, God. How did I hit my head? Why am I on the floor? I must have passed out. This is a nightmare I'm not waking up from. I can't wake up from him.

He smacks my cheeks. "Danny! Speak to me!" His dank, graveyard breath fogs over me. He scours my eyes like he's trying to read the name on a headstone.

This must be how Starky felt when the TV started talking to him.

7:06 AM: "Sheeit!" Officer Beef bounds into the jail cell.

Thank God he's finally here. I cry. Relief. Grief. Confusion. The whole night rains out of me in torrents.

Captain leaps from my side to make room for Officer Beef. Captain apologizes, "It happened so fast, Officer! His eyes rolled back in his head! Then he fell straight to the floor — I tried — but I couldn't catch him in time!"

Officer Beef drops next to me, smelling like a coffee shop from heaven. "Sheeit!" He shines a pen-light in my eyes. He flicks it off. "Ya know where y'are, son?"

"Jail." My tears sop down the sides of my cheeks filling the pot holes of my ears. "Doing my time, like you are, Officer."

"Very good."

"No one is watching me on a videotape, are they?!" I bolt up and dig my fingers into his arm so he won't leave me again. "My signature doesn't mean anything on the contract I signed, does it? And I'm not taking over anyone's perch? I'm getting out of here in one hour and I'm done! Right?!" A worm of snot curls out of my nose.

"Yer paperwork is in now." Officer whips a hanky out of his pocket.

He wipes up my face. I hold his wrists, "No one will be watching me, will they?!"

"Not after ya get released." Like I'm an invalid, he gently boosts me up to the wall so I can rest my back.

"I earned Happy Time?"

"Take it easy. How many fingers am I holdin' up?" He holds up four pudgy fingers.

Captain squats next to him. He holds up four skeleton-like fingers and murmurs in between them. "Why the number four? Is it because that's the number of points I missed on the bar exam? Why not three fingers? The Father, Son, and the Holy Spirit."

I nod toward Captain and whisper to Beef, "Tell him to stop! He's scaring me."

Beefy wrenches out of my grasp to put the gooey hanky in his breast pocket. "Firs', tell me how many fingers ya see."

Captain warns, "It's a trick question. He might revoke your Happy Time. Keep you here another five days."

I look from one to the other. "Is it a trick question?"

"Nope. No right answer. Just need ta know whachoo see."

Captain exhales loudly, "Bar exam was full of questions where you can't give a straight answer."

Officer Beef says, "Focus! Can ya focus on me?" I focus on his beautiful, fat face. "Jus' do yer best. Tell me how many fingers ya see."

I nod to both of their four-fingers. "You mean total?"

"Total."

I guess, "Eight?"

Captain smacks his forehead. "Infinity, Danny!"

Officer peels my fingers off his arm. He gets up. "Double vision. I hafta check with a doctor."

I snatch his pant leg. "You can't leave me alone with him any longer! It's his fault I fell on my head! Don't go!"

Beef squints at me, surprised. "Is that what all this fuss is about?" He kneels down and takes my shoulders in his hands. "You're having a bad trip, young man."

"How come you didn't come in here all night long? Not even one time! Why didn't you stop him?"

"Stop who?" Beef's expression changes.

I point to Captain. "Him!"

Beef pats my white-knuckled hand. "There's no one else in here."

"What?!" Captain and I shout in unison.

I repeatedly point to Captain who clambers up. "He's right THERE!"

"There's no one but you." Beef stretches in front of my face, blocking me from seeing Captain. "Hey. Yew've been all alone here. All night long. I checked in a…" He takes a piece of paper out of his breast pocket and reads, "Kirk Anderson."

Captain hushes, "Oh, God. Oh, God."

Beef waves the paper in front of my face. "Mr. Anderson? Thas' your name? Y'all need to stay with me."

I snap back to Officer. "Yes. That's me. I'm him. I'm Kirk Anderson."

"Okay. One Kirk Anderson was checked in. One Kirk Anderson is bein' released at 8:00 AM. Anybody else will stay locked up in this cell forever. In purgatory. I'll make sure he never gits out. Okay?" Officer Beef pushes up his own large girth. "Now y'all sit tight."

I catapult after him. Spread my arms. Block him. "Don't go!"

He frowns with his chin out. "Mr. Anderson, you need to move aside."

"Please! Take me with you!"

Beef pokes a finger in my chest. "Y'all are jus' 'bout outta here. Now listen to me. Yew can pull it together. Or yew can keep this up and I will be forced to request a psych evaluation which will delay yer release."

"No, no, no delay!" I recede and put my hands up. "I'll pull it together!"

Officer Beef shakes his head and waddles out. *SLAM!*

He's gone. Gone for forty-seven minutes. Thirteen minutes have passed after the hour. Thirteen is an unlucky number. Whole buildings are built without that floor. But seven is lucky. The numbers are giving me contradictory messages. I turn back around.

To Kirk.

7:13 AM: I swallow; "Are you me?"

"It fucking looks like it."

"You're Kirk Anderson?"

"Yes."

"You said your name was Captain."

"Captain KIRK! Are you retarded?" He flings his bony arm at me. "What about you? I knew Danny Johnson was a bullshit name."

"I'm not going to be YOU!! I'm not going to be John the Baptist!"

"Oh yeah? What makes you think you can escape? This is your fate! They've already snapped your nose in their trap."

I denounce, “You’re nothing but a bad trip. The guard said so! I’m not talking to you.” I scurry into my corner and make myself as small as a mouse.

“We are the same person — we look exactly the same!”

“Fuck you! I don’t look like you!” He looks like human remains, not like me.

“That’s why I was so scared when you woke me up — I saw myself — but myself as a teenager — standing right in front of me. Me! Exactly!” He bends down to me. His cloudy pupils look into mine like he’s looking in a mirror. “I assumed you saw we are identical. It’s so obvious.”

I shove him. He skids on his haunches but keeps talking, “I didn’t know what you were — an angel? But of me. All night long, the only thing that made sense to me was that you were my clone. That the CIA made you and planned this. But, to be honest, what I hoped for was you were maybe a son I didn’t know I had. That’s why I asked what your mother’s name is. What is it, by the way? Really.”

I stare hard at the floor. “Crawl back in your coffin, man. I mean it!”

He inches toward me. “Georgia? Right? We’re the same person, kid. Father is Bill. Rory, Helen and Celia are our sisters.”

Was Starky able to change the channel on his TV? Or would it keep talking to him even if he turned it off?

Captain Kirk’s only in my head. I just have to find a way to unplug him.

7:34 AM: What was in that pot? It’s horrible. I’ll never sneak into Steve’s brother’s stash again. My hallucinations will be gone once I get out of here and I can go home and take care of myself. My mom will feel sorry for me. She’ll make me a stew with biscuits and her homemade raspberry jam. I’ll detox. Turn on my lava lamp and sleep eighteen hours straight in my very own bed.

It will feel so good waking up tomorrow in my own room: the sun streaming in through my window, smelling waffles and bacon. My sisters playing *Dreamboat Annie* too loudly. I'll lie there thinking about this night. I'll laugh.

Then again, I won't laugh. Nothing about this is funny. Earlier, I thought I'd share the tale of my night in jail with my buddies the next time we lit up. But I won't. How could I actually believe that I — the golden boy of the family — could ever live the horror Captain Kirk described? Christ, I'd rather die. No. No one, ever, will find out how close I came to losing my mind tonight.

It's now my second darkly held secret. Two darkly held secrets? That means a third one is coming. Because Bad Things Come in Threes. Like smoking laced pot, hallucinating all night, and landing on my head.

What's next?

His putrid vapors waft over me. He's so real. I just touched him. I swear I did.

It's entirely possible that Beefcake pretended not to see Captain Kirk. Beefy had a lousy attitude with me when I was admitted last night. He wanted me to learn a lesson. They could be mounting this exact same fright show with every kid who gets busted for drugs and thrown in the slammer.

In fact, this cell could be a special teenagers' holding cell where the government tries to scare us, its youth and future, away from drugs. This could totally be a CIA program. It makes sense. Because what would happen to Social Security if a whole generation is too stoned to pay into the system? They need us to earn money! We have to pay for their retirement and benefits, so they can stay at home and watch TV.

Or this is like in the military, where I hear they aim to break down the individual. Its overdone method of *Scare the*

Shit out of the Teenager Who Otherwise Has So Much Potential is obviously another way of trying to break my spirit. Keeping me from expressing myself. Any judge would gladly sign off on this charade so the government can con me. Beefy and Captain must both be highly trained actors. They each received special briefings on me when I was getting my jumpsuit. This is all one big scam. A hidden camera *Twilight Zone* for troubled teens, which I'm not.

"I should be the one to get out. Not you." Captain Kirk says sideways.

I shoot back, "Shut the fuck up."

7:41 AM: I close my eyes. Cover my ears. But his voice ghosts inside my head, "I figured something out over the last nine minutes and thirty seconds. It's your fault I wound up living under a freeway."

Clenching my eyes tighter, a vision of Captain Kirk appears in my brain. Like I'm pushing my nose through a scratchy bush, spying on him in his dark bedroom at night. Except it's not a bedroom. He's hunched underneath a freeway. Rain's dripping all around him. A flicker from a lighter illuminates his face as he inhales off a pipe. Crumbled crackers are next to him.

Captain Kirk continues, "It wasn't the CIA. It was you. I see it so clearly now. Like when you trace your steps backward looking for something you lost. I found what I was looking for. And it was you."

Close my eyes tighter. No more! I don't want to see him and how he lives. But, no matter how hard I will against it, an infestation of sights swarms through my mind.

This time they're of me: I see me, eight years old, in my scout's uniform skimming cash from my mom's wallet. Stealing gum. Stealing toy cars. Then I'm nine, opening our medicine cabinet. Guzzling cough syrup. I'm fourteen and I'm night skiing: smoking my first joint on the not double date. Lynette and I share a bong, parked in the family station wagon. The police tapping on the window. Lynette breaking up with me over the phone. Joss and I sharing Madanuska Thunderfuck on a bunk, smiling from ear to ear. Steve and I hot dog off ski jumps. We share a joint on the chair lift. As a busboy, cleaning up after my shift, drinking leftover Sangria. I'm blowing pot smoke outside my bedroom window and doing my homework. My friends and I break into a storage container and steal a keg of beer. It's a sunny day in the park and we're smoking a joint while we're throwing a frisbee.

Captain Kirk's voice vibrates my core, "You're having fun now. Except for Lynette. But the real pain is later. And guess who comes later? I do! I pay for it. Not you. Your actions are my consequences. You FUCK!"

I cringe and spy at him. His ashy knuckles cover his eyes. "Yes, this is your fault. You set the path for me. I'm locked in here forever for what you did. What you're going to do…." His face twists, he sobs. His mouth stretches open like a mummy in a museum.

I cover my head to stop the pictures from coming. But they wiggle through my arms and show me more: I see me and Joss at the University of Washington. He passes me a baggie of weed as we enter a lecture hall. A joint sticking in between my teeth as I'm writing a paper. My professor peers over his glasses at me, returning it. The grade is a C minus. Me and Joss approach a group of co-eds with joints over our ears. I'm interning in an office: an employee offers me LSD. I slip it in my pocket. Walking away after a study group at USC, I light up. Studying in my apartment alone, I take a toke. I open my girlfriend's closet to see it's emptied of all her clothes. I ride in a passenger seat, the sleazy attorney slams into reverse, crashing into another car. On Santa Monica beach, I study for the bar, gazing at the sun and the ladies. I take the California Bar Exam.

Get drunk with a lady on the plane. Snort coke while studying for the bar in Washington. I run into Lynette outside Denny's. Lynette drinks, I snort with her stepbrother. Lynette buys her own engagement ring. Lynette holds her hand over her abdomen. I work in a t-shirt factory and snort coke. I work in a video dating service and snort coke with the owner. I ignore bills in the mail. Mom gives me money. I mainline coke and see a UFO. I steal my mom's jewelry and sell it at a pawn shop. I can't find a vein in my arm to mainline. Mom buys me a car. I sell it for crack. Mom buys me another car. I sell it for crack. Mom refuses to give me more money. I get evicted from my own apartment and look for places to sleep outside. Conspiracy numbers are everywhere. Dash across the freeway. Secret codes come from lights and license plates. Pull a tooth out of my mouth. Sleep under the freeway. Sleep over hot air vents. Sit on my perch and deal drugs. Wash under my arms in a public park restroom. Get a baggie of crack from White. Smile at her kid who hugs his lunch. Smoke crack behind a dumpster. Walk in the rain and hide my face from the CIA. Stand in line at a soup kitchen. Going bald in places but the rest of my hair is long. Nails long. Face dirty. Clothes are hard as cardboard. Under the overpass, it's dark and raining. I hunch on my sleeping bag while inhaling from a crack pipe. Rats peek at me from underneath the blackberry bushes. They scurry to my crackers. Tracing blue lights shimmer off their tails.

Jesus. How was I supposed to know those little things added up?

Captain Kirk is here with me now. I know it. Maybe it's just the guard who is the highly-trained actor getting paid to act like he doesn't see Captain Kirk. Or could it be that God has given me a special gift? Maybe that's it. Maybe only I can see Captain Kirk because God wants it that way. But I know for certain Captain Kirk is real.

Watching him cry, it feels like a rat is biting into my heart. I can't unclench its jaws or tear it away. I could smother it with a good, deep toke. But, obviously, I can't do that now. The only way to stop the piercing pain is to make Captain Kirk stop crying.

I plead, "I'm sorry it turned out like that. I'm serious."

If only I could change things. I would give anything just to give him a normal life. He ignores me. Sunk, I pick up the kites and the pencil nubs.

What can I do now? There isn't a do-over. I can't undo what he's done to himself.

Can I?

7:52 AM: Eight minutes left. Infinity. Seven fifty-two. Twenty-six times two. Two is for second chances. That's it! A second chance in life. I'll go completely straight. I offer, "What if we're here because we're being given another chance? To do it right."

Captain Kirk hangs his head. "I told you not to bullshit a bullshitter. You're not changing. I know you."

"No. Captain." I stand firm. "I will do everything right."

"Liar."

"Okay. Yes, I've lied. But I'm not now. There's no way I will live the future I just saw! I refuse. I don't want that for either of us. I'm telling you, I'll go straight today!"

He unrolls enough toilet paper to mummify his whole body. "Whatever. If it makes you feel better."

"Look, I can't change what I've done already. But college and law school I can do something about. It's not too late for that. You know I'm right."

"If only."

"No, Captain, listen! I think — I truly think, God is giving you and me a second chance! Why couldn't this crazy night be His miracle? You could wake up tomorrow and your life could be completely different! It could be! I mean, you and me meeting is a weird warp in time. So why don't we take advantage of it?!"

With quiet realization, he says, "Yes, it could be a miracle."

"I will straighten up! I promise you, man. I swear on my life, I'll never do any drugs ever again! Ever! I'll study — I won't mess around — I'll do everything — so you can — I can…No, I WILL be a lawyer. And I'll have, you'll have, a house, with a wife and kids. Take them on ski vacations. Can't you see it? I believe it's going to happen. Because I don't want a life of purgatory! I've changed. You've changed me. I've changed forever."

"Yes." His eyes fill with hope. "You could be right. This is an opportunity. A second chance." He stands.

"I won't disappoint you again." The biting on my heart softens. It works. Just the decision to change makes me feel better already.

He nods, "What time is it now?" I turn around, one last time, to look in the guard's station.

7:58 AM: The hand ticks two minutes closer to my new life. Beef is on the phone, writing in a folder. Our eyes meet. I nod, assuring him I'm not crazy. He nods back at me and closes what is probably my file. Guess that means there won't be a psych evaluation. I can't deal with one extra minute between me and my freedom. I'm on my way to being a new man.

BAM! Captain Kirk pounds his fist in my ear. I fly — my head bashes on the wall. My whole head reverberates. My knees crumble. The room whirls. I collapse. I'm unable to move from the gonging pain. Captain Kirk straddles my chest. His cold, bony hands clamp down on my neck. They tighten like a vise. I pry them. I can't breathe. "*AGH!*"

His graveyard breath fumes on me. "Even if you could scream, he thinks you're hallucinating. No one's coming back for ninety-nine seconds."

"*GHUH!*" There's a nub on the floor somewhere. My hand flops around for it. Just cement. I'm slipping under the manhole again, where no one can hear me.

Through his cigarette butts, he scowls. "This second chance isn't ours, you idiot! It's MINE! I'm taking over!"

The flood ferrets through my veins with its furry warmth, seducing me. I want to float peacefully away from this nightmare. It would be so easy to flush away from my problems with its gushing, comforting, tide. No — I can't pass out again — I'll die!

I resurface. His thorny-veined eyes drill into mine. He hisses, "Which wolf lives? Not a trick question. The one you feed." He shakes my neck, "And. You. Fed. Me!"

My fingertip finds a nub. Snatch it. Swing it. Jab his eye. His hands fly to his face. "*AHHHH!!*"

Wheezing, I stumble up. A mouse released from its trap. Coughing, I use the bench to stand. Swing the nub at his other eye. He screams, "*AAGHHH!!!*"

I hurl him back. Push his head on the floor. Straddle his chest. He cries out and covers his eyes.

Grab kites. Stuff them. Cut my knuckles on his teeth. Bury his fucking kites in the urn that is his throat. I shove it all back. Conspiracy. His perch. Mistakes. Pot. Crack. CIA. Lynette. Law School. The Masons. Down his tomb. He convulses.

No more kites. I shake his neck like he shook mine. Bang his skull. He's not moving.

Captain Kirk is dead and I am free.

I tried to help him. It's his own fault.

The cell door opens. Officer Beef calls my name. MY NAME! Not his! Not his name anymore!

I go toward Officer Beef. Must act normal. Like nothing happened.

8:08 AM: Infinity two times. Is there such a thing?

My eyes sting. It's the sun. Rare — a sunny day in Seattle. Is there a rainbow?

My clothes feel good on me. I pat my list which is in my front pocket. Hell behind me. I survived and I'm stronger because I defeated my demon. There's the rainbow: God's promise. It will never be all rain again because there's hope, and I found the pot of gold. This new chance at life is my very own pot of gold.

Steve's Mercedes reflects the sunlight. It blinds me as he pulls up. The bass from his pulsing speakers hurts my whole body. How can I ask him to turn it down? Steve pushes open the passenger side door — my head throbs with the blare of the music.

He leans across the seat. Seeing me, his face falls. Then he cracks up. He turns the volume way down. "Oh fuck! Dude! You look like shit!"

I snort. Hell, he must be right. Must be funny.

He snickers, "Get in! Get in!" I get inside. Close the door. Love this car. It makes me feel like a rock star. What a way to leave jail!

Steve jerks it into gear and rips out. I'm thrown back in my seat. He makes a goofy face and smacks the steering wheel. "What the fuck happened to you?"

"Need — aspirin." My throat is swollen, I can barely talk. "My head."

Steve swerves around an old building. He pulls his sunglasses down and spot checks the premises. He slips a joint out of his breast pocket. "Better than aspirin!" He lights it up and takes a long hit. Through his sucked-in breath he says, "This will help your head."

The smoke swirls right into my nostrils. Thai Stick. Oh, God. It is so, so good. But I turn away. What do I say? What's my excuse? I won't do any drugs with him ever again. But I'll never, ever, tell him the real reason why. My throat raw, I etch out, "I had a really bad trip. It was so real."

Steve exhales, "Nooooooooooo!" He shakes his head with great sympathy. "Hair o' the dog. Calm that shit down." The car fills with the velvety smoke. My head is floating in his cloud and I want to linger in it. But I'm done with drugs. Forever.

Steve holds the joint out to me.

I turn my head and roll down my window. No way. No how.

Then again, I already breathed in Steve's second hand smoke.

I take the damn joint. It will definitely help my head. After what I went through, I deserve to be free of pain. Plus, I'll sleep longer, and will wake up, rested, tomorrow morning.

That's when I'll start my new life. Tomorrow.

I inhale.

"Infinity."

What the fuck was that—? I spin around.

I see Captain Kirk in the back seat. He half-smiles at me, crosses his legs, and turns to gaze out the window.

The End

The authors would greatly appreciate
an honest review on Amazon.

For more information about drugs and mental illness
please go to: http://www.ANightInJail.com

To hear a song which was inspired by this book, go to

"I Know Where I'm Going"
by
Connor Swan Smith
https://soundcloud.com/connor-swan-smith/
i-know-where-im-going